the Full Diet

the Full Diet

A Weight-Loss Doctor's 7-Day Guide to Shedding Pounds for Good

Michael A. Snyder, M.D., F.A.C.S.

HAY HOUSE, INC.
Carlsbad, California • New York City
London • Sydney • Johannesburg
Vancouver • Hong Kong • New Delhi

Published and distributed in the United States by: Hay House, Inc.: www .hayhouse.com • *Published and distributed in Australia by:* Hay House Australia Pty. Ltd.: www.hayhouse.com.au • *Published and distributed in the United Kingdom by:* Hay House UK, Ltd.: www.hayhouse.co.uk • *Published and distributed in the Republic of South Africa by:* Hay House SA (Pty), Ltd.: www.hayhouse.co.za • *Distributed in Canada by:* Raincoast: www.raincoast. com • *Published in India by:* Hay House Publishers India: www.hayhouse.co.in

Design: Jami Goddess • *Interior illustrations:* Black Top Design

The hardcover edition of this book was published under the title *Full: A Life Without Dieting*

The Library of Congress has cataloged the hardcover edition as follows:

Snyder, Michael A.
 Full : a life without dieting ; weight-loss secrets from a weight-loss surgeon (without the surgery!) / Michael A. Snyder. -- 1st ed.
     p. cm.
 ISBN 978-1-4019-2905-3 (hardcover : alk. paper) 1. Weight loss. I. Title.
 RM222.2.S634 2011
 613.2'5--dc22

                              2010029888

Tradepaper ISBN: 978-1-4019-2906-0
Digital ISBN: 978-1-4019-4037-9

15 14 13 12   5 4 3 2
1st edition, December 2010
2nd edition, May 2012

Printed in the United States of America

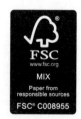

To my patients, who teach me every day about the wonders of the body as well as the practical secrets to successful weight loss. Their stories, struggles, and experiences are what challenge me to be a better physician; and their faith in me inspires me to be a better person. I feel honored that they trust me to take care of them and enlist me as a partner in a most intimate quest: to improve their health and their lives. Without their insights, integrity, and courage, this book would not be possible.

I also dedicate this book to those who have grappled with weight issues. I am constantly reminded that virtually everyone struggles with weight, and, in the grander picture, with self-confidence and happiness. This book is for you.

Contents

Introduction

THE FULL STORY: ONE DOCTOR'S MISSION TO END ALL DIETING— AND THE MISERY THAT GOES WITH IT

Never diet again. Ever.

That has been my motto since I first became a weight-loss surgeon and suddenly found myself witnessing the effects of traditional dieting on people who struggle their whole lives trying to lose weight. I've always said that "never dieting again" is the short answer to the seemingly bewildering question of what we should do to lose excess weight permanently and be optimally healthy, whether we're trying to shed hundreds of pounds or just those last and furious 15. I wrote the first edition to this book based on this precept.

But then something happened. I realized that just because I was promoting the antidiet didn't mean I couldn't offer a defined program. The word "diet," after all, simply refers to a way of eating. In this regard, my book is indeed a diet. I also realized that people desperately want a program—an explicit set of rules and strategies they can apply to their lives. So yes, this is a diet, but it's not the traditional diet of cutting calories or eliminating foods. It's a program that will help ease you into a new way of eating. A way that will still be filled with the joy of food.

In my surgery practice, I care for morbidly obese patients every day who resort to surgery to gain control of their weight. But over the past few years, since starting my company Fullbar, my life has become equally filled with people who are not candidates for surgery and who simply need to lose 5 to 80 or so pounds. In this regard, I'm a source of advice and encouragement for people whose anatomy I never touch yet whose challenges can be just as epic as those who opt for surgery. And those are the people for whom this book can really make a difference. The groups of people I've taken through my out-of-the-operating-room program have proven how powerful the strategies in this book can be; you'll even meet and see the victories of many of these people as you read through these pages.

I'm going to take you on a journey using what I've gleaned from my practice and my experiences with Fullbar to maximize your weight-loss experience and get you to embark on a "diet" like you've never done before. I lay out a specific program designed to help you gain lasting control of your waistline, but more important, I provide all the information you need to know to live a full yet slim life without ever going on a traditional diet again.

I'll be honest: just because I'm giving you an explicit program doesn't mean it will be as easy as 1-2-3, and it does require that you actually *do* something. But what I'm about to show you is so simple that even you can handle—and master—it, and I don't care where you're coming from. Maybe you're someone who has failed every attempt to permanently lose weight. Maybe you hate to exercise and believe food is the enemy. Maybe your picture is next to the definition of *emotional eater* in the dictionary. Maybe you've got so much weight to lose that you're contemplating bariatric surgery. And maybe you don't have all that much to drop (those "last ten pounds") but would just like to stop obsessing about calories, belly fat, and what you put into your mouth on a daily basis. No matter what your personal circumstances are, I've probably seen—and dealt with—it among the thousands of people I've encountered and patients I've treated. Even if the thought of being happy with your weight and losing the excess pounds *without dieting* seems impossible and you don't even want to try, I want you to at least take this book seriously. You might think you're unlike any other person out there looking to lose weight, but I'm going to prove you wrong.

Let me say one thing, right from the start: I'd love nothing more than to put myself out of business. On most days, I can be found in a chilly, dimly lit operating room. I stare at a pair of flat-screen monitors positioned to float above the head of my anesthetized patient. The image I view is captured from a scope that I have passed all the way through the patient's abdominal wall. I am constantly manipulating staplers, graspers, burning devices, and scissors at the end of very long instruments that enable me to perform surgeries. I attach adjustable, restrictive, gastric bands or bypass lengths of small bowel to stomachs that I have dramatically reduced in size. I do these routine procedures 14 to 20 times per week, totaling more than 3,500 times to date. And, as you might imagine, there is no shortage of work for me. By the time you read this, the combined weight lost will have totaled more than 200,000 pounds.

All that I just described is done in an effort to give my patients an advantage over their genetics and their habits. You see, if you are morbidly obese—on average, about 100 pounds or more overweight—you are at a distinct disadvantage. There is less than a 5 percent chance that you can lose weight and keep it off. This has been proven by no less than the National Institutes of Health. So that is why my bariatric surgery practice exists. I want to give my patients a fighting chance.

But what does this mean if you're not in this category of severely overweight people? You have much less weight to lose, and you are probably not in as poor medical health as my patients who suffer from dangerously high blood pressure or type 2 diabetes as a result of their weight. Your advantage may be your genetics, your activity level, or your dietary habits. But still, nearly everyone thinks about his or her weight. Do you know anyone who doesn't? I didn't think so.

What you can learn from me is what my patients have to share. Like you, they have lost the same ten or more pounds a countless number of times, but they haven't resigned themselves to a lifetime of cyclic dieting and on-again, off-again programs. They've left that world far behind because they know it takes more than desire and willpower to win this battle. Instead, they have discovered the true secret to permanent weight control: a simple set of practical tools that can be tailored to their lifestyle and personal choices and which allows them to do things like "cheat" on junk food and enjoy a buffet table. I've acquired these tools through my practice and now pass them on to you. What my patients have learned in making these tools work for them and sustaining their weight-loss goals—without a Herculean effort—is what this book is about. The challenges they have faced, as well as the triumphs they have achieved, are all valuable lessons that anyone can use to his or her own weight-loss advantage.

My patients have already been through the process of feeling really bad about themselves. What's more, they've been humbled to the point of acknowledging that diets don't work because diets are beyond their control. Diets are too fragile—they make it too easy to fail. Think about yourself: Haven't all of your previous efforts relied upon desire and willpower to no avail? How many times have you felt that "if you just had more self-control" you'd be able to manage your weight better? Or, "maybe it's not important enough for me" to win this battle? Well, I'd counter that it *is* terribly important to you and that perhaps you have done more to win this fight than just about anything else you've done in your life. And I bet the battle has gone on for decades. You've no doubt put significant time, money, and real pain into the process.

So again, I reiterate: It's not all about heart, desire, and willpower. Rather, it's about finding and utilizing simple and realistic tools to change your life. Like my patients, you need to find such real tools that will fit into your life without the pain, inhuman effort, and disappointment. It's about being realistic and recognizing what your personal, real potential is. The goal is not for me to set out a program telling you exactly what you should do. And I don't want you to believe you have to become an expert on the chemistry of metabolism, good carbs versus bad carbs, and so on, to lose weight. That's just crazy! I'm going to make you an expert at figuring out what will work for you. Period. All I care about is your personal experience.

The vast majority of the population has it all wrong when they look at morbidly obese individuals and pass judgment. As you'll learn through this book, my patients are cursed by their DNA. They cannot win the weight battle despite their best efforts. But after surgery, they are on the same playing field as everyone else. The weight-loss and maintenance tools that work for the average person can finally work for them, but they still have to apply those tools. Surgery is not a quick fix that lasts forever. The heart of my practice is not performing procedures. It's what we do once my patients recover and embrace a new digestive process and a new way of life. It's in teaching my patients how to succeed *afterward*. I like to say that having the surgery is like getting married. The actual getting-married part is easy; staying married, well, that's another thing entirely!

I'm certain that the same principles I teach my gastric bypass and band patients to maintain their success (and watch their weight get lower and lower and lower) can help everyone else, too. Including you. No unrealistic deprivations required. No fasting, detoxing, exhaustive point or calorie counting, or two-week "fast track" dieting that sheds some initial water weight only to return later with a vengeance.

Unlike most diet books, *The Full Diet* shares my secrets about how we are wired and how we process the required changes (that is, how our minds work in weight-management efforts). What's more, most traditional diet books perpetuate the problem, plunging people deeper into obsessions with food and weight, which lead to rebounds and more weight gain, rather than genuinely helping people establish healthier habits for a lifetime. After all, when we look at the statistics (explored in detail in Chapter 1), the more diet books and weight-loss ideas that get put out there, the fatter we seem to get.

No day passes without an advertisement for yet another tip to losing weight; and no month passes without another diet book hitting bookshelves touting something "revolutionary." Our desire to read about losing weight is surpassed only by our desire to try doing so. We spend more than $55 billion a year on weight-loss programs and diets. And yet the results of all that dieting continue to be bleak. In 2009, a report published by researchers at Emory University and sponsored by the United Health Foundation and the American Public Health Association put it bluntly: by 2018, the United States could expect to spend $344 billion on health-care costs attributable to obesity, and would account for a whopping 21 percent of health-care spending—up from 9.1 percent today. Between 1990 and today, obesity rates have doubled, and obesity now accounts for one-third of the increase in our nation's health-care costs. There are more obese individuals in this country than those who are merely overweight. Why can't all these weight-loss ideas help reverse the trend? Something is profoundly missing. There is a huge disconnect between the notion of losing weight and actually doing it. This book will help you to resolve that disconnect within yourself once and for all.

I am constantly being asked my opinion on popular diet programs, especially when they are new. I am implored to legitimate any number of the fast and trendy programs, drugs, hormone-stimulating products, and/or membership-driven start-ups. My answer always starts the same way. "If this were really such a big deal and truly the 'last word' on how to control your weight, don't you think you'd be reading about it on page one of *The New York Times*? Don't you think that the real 'ultimate weight-loss solution' would not be one that you had to wade through the Internet to find? Don't you think it would already be at hand and celebrated coast to coast?"

Throw out the claims you have been promised. Stop the process now before it ruins your faith in your potential. Start being realistic and listen to how I can give the power back to you.

A Little about Me

To start, I grew up in Miami and wanted nothing more than to be an archaeologist and world traveler. (I was really affected by the *Indiana Jones* movie series!) I later ended up at Harvard University, where I received a degree in anthropology with a focus on archaeology. I knew that I wanted to work the world over, and thought I could best do that as a doctor. I had this fantasy about digging in the dirt and taking care of the people. Never tell a 22-year-old that he cannot do everything. So I returned to Miami and got my medical degree from the University of Miami School of Medicine. Then I went on to Oregon Health Sciences University to become a general surgeon, thinking I'd focus on trauma.

But mastering laparoscopic surgery and getting a peek into the world of gastric bypass surgery during a two-year tour of duty in Virginia shifted the course of my future. I was amazed by bariatric surgery, which helps people achieve healthy weights through surgery. It is reserved for a specific class of overweight people: those whose weight has reached a level where it negatively impacts their health. If you understand body mass index, or BMI, you know that bariatric surgery is for those whose BMI is greater than or equal to 35. BMI is a simple calculation of height and weight ratio. A BMI of less than 25 is the goal for most people, but different BMIs are acceptable, depending on your body shape and type.

I quickly left the world of appendectomies and the ER to answer my calling in bariatrics where I could participate in people's journeys to conquering severe obesity. The enriching relationships I forged in bariatrics far outshined those I had experienced in other specialties that rarely saw such dramatic results and hard-won transformations. Saving the life of a person in the emergency room is one thing, but being able to coach from the ringside as people face the weight that has beaten up their bodies and their lives is another. To this day, I feel like a long-term partner in the lives of my patients rather than just a doctor with a certain specialty who drops in to save the day in a singular moment.

I've been fortunate to have learned and mastered the latest bariatric techniques from the pioneers in the field who have truly catapulted this medical specialty from a somewhat primitive state decades ago to a highly advanced practice now. Denver Bariatrics opened its doors in 2000, and has been nationally recognized as a Center of Excellence by the American Society for Metabolic and Bariatric Surgery. Most of my patients also have some of the medical problems associated with obesity, such as depression, reflux, diabetes, high blood pressure, high lipids (cholesterol and/or triglycerides), menstrual irregularity, infertility, urinary stress incontinence, sleep apnea (disordered sleep), and joint pain. Bariatric surgery, ultimately, is not about weight. It's about the weight's effect on the person's health. When someone is called "morbidly obese," he has reached a point where his weight has adverse effects on his health. It is never a comment about a patient's appearance or value as a person. It's very important to understand that it is not a judgment about the person. It's about the patient's health.

After a few years at the clinic, I came to realize that there was a gap in what I could provide to people. Not everyone qualifies for surgery, yet everyone wants to feel satisfied at meals, happy with their weight, and healthy. I was working hard to help the morbidly obese, but not for everyone else. A close friend of mine said, "I get what you're doing for your morbidly obese patients, but what do you have for my aunt who cannot lose 30 pounds and is suffering from many life and health issues because of it?" It was unacceptable that I had nothing for her. That had to change, which has led not only to my forays into developing an international food supplementation company, but also to the book you're holding in your hands.

Now about You

You cannot live a full life if you think about weight constantly, or if weight issues have become the bane of your existence. I've spent my career and much of my own energy taking care of weight issues. Don't let my current "normal-sized" physique fool you: I've struggled with my own weight problems in the past and this has given me an intimate knowledge of how such concerns affect people's health, life, longevity, and self-esteem. Granted, I've never been morbidly obese nor needed bariatric surgery, but I know what it's like to struggle with weight and let it take control of everything. What I didn't learn from my own weight issues I've discovered through my patients. As with so many of my patients, if you can come to live a full life and be happy with the weight your body achieves after taking my techniques to heart, then I will have considered my mission complete.

Have your past dieting efforts been a series of attempts to

white-knuckle it through every experience, whether it's fighting the buffet table at a party or avoiding taboo foods at a baseball game? Has it always been about what you *cannot* put into your body to gain control? If so, then you know that you're very good for a period of time, then kind of good. Then you begin to slack off, and eventually enough slacking off happens for you to forget the whole endeavor.

Not only is that process bad for you physiologically but it also affects how you feel about yourself. Nowhere else in your life do you allow this predictable and dependable cycle of repeated failure. What if your work life went this way? How many failures would it take before you were fired or demoted? How about in your personal relationships? What if you were 92 percent monogamous? How many infidelities would it take for your significant other to leave? And what if you were careful with your toddler "most" of the time? How long would it take until Child Protective Services came to take your child from you?

In my opinion there are three things in my patients' lives that change them forever: getting married, having children, and undergoing bariatric surgery. Maybe your list is similar. Of course, there are many other things that can change you pretty quickly, such as winning the lottery, getting divorced, going through personal bankruptcy, and losing a loved one. But for argument's sake, I think marriage, children, and bariatric surgery rank somewhere near the top. In a single moment, any of these events dramatically shifts your life.

None of these undertakings is to be entered upon lightly. They entail big obligations. They involve relationships that require a lifetime of vigilance and nurturing. Most of us wouldn't compromise our efforts with a spouse or a child. When things are important to you, no amount of work is too much to make them a success. Until you approach your health in the same way, you'll never achieve the same success. This is what I talk about when I say it's got to matter to you. It's true that losing 20 pounds doesn't have the same implication as being a bad parent. But you get my point. This is one of the primary secrets to maintaining a healthy weight, so I'll be reiterating it throughout the book.

The Full Promise

As the subtitle says, this is a seven-day guide to weight loss. Am I really promising results in seven days? Well, yes and no.

Here's the deal: I've structured this program over the course of seven days because you can learn everything you really need to know about how to lose weight in that short amount of time. Losing the weight takes effort and willpower, but knowing *how* shouldn't be hard at all.

Each of the main seven chapters is written to provide you with information that will help you understand various issues associated with weight loss. At the end of each of these chapters, I give you specific things to do that are based on the information you just read—this is the "program" of the book.

My suggestion is that you read one chapter each day, and really take in the information. Think about it. Think about how it applies to your life and your weight-loss goals. Working with the information and making it personal will increase your chances of lasting success. But if you don't want to read this book in seven days, take as much or as little time as you need. Plan it out over the course of a month if you like. Take two days to read each chapter and see where you are two weeks from now. Or read it all in one sitting and apply as many strategies as you can today, tomorrow, the next day, and so on. Do what works best for you.

So what is the Full promise? My promise to you is that if you take just one of my recommendations seriously, you will see results in a matter of days. It might not be serious pounds on the scale, but you will *feel* different. You will be breaking new ground in your body's journey to a healthier, sustainable weight. Then, just that singular sensation of knowing that you're doing *something* will inspire you to keep going . . . and to incorporate another strategy into your life. Soon enough, you'll be on the fast track to significant results. And best of all, you'll know how to keep going or at least how to maintain what you've accomplished.

Remember, this isn't like other diets you've ever been on. I'm teaching you a lifestyle. I'm showing you how to deal with the reality of our eating habits in a manner that honors your body's needs while allowing you to simultaneously make minimal shifts in how you've already been living. I realize that change is hard. It's just not human nature to make major changes overnight, much less over any period of time if those changes amount to a radical reversal of ingrained behaviors. So let's take this one step, and one day at a time.

In This Book

In this book, you will not find an inflexible set meal plan or daily regimen. You can continue to eat whatever you normally eat while applying specific strategies that will help you to gain better control over your sense of fullness—without feeling deprived or restricted. That said, you will find plenty of structure in the tools I offer, so there's no confusion or sense that you are left to your own insatiable devices.

For those who really need a meal plan, I've got a one-month list of ideas for you to consider, as well as a way to commence a fast-track "induction" phase to get the weight loss happening rapidly. The people whose successes are featured throughout this book all went through a version of this program, and they all took part in the Induction Phase. It helped them accelerate their journey, set the tone for their new lifestyle habits, and extinguish certain cravings that dominated their previous eating behaviors. Although these participants relied on Fullbar products to help them, the program outlined in this book can generate the same results without any of these products. You will learn doable strategies and tools that you can incorporate into your daily life. These don't depend on any single food item, restriction, or rigid regimen, and they have helped hundreds of people find success with weight loss.

For those who struggle immensely with portion control, finding high-quality products to boost their weight loss, and getting thrown off course by inconvenience, you may want to check out the options at www.fullbar.com. These products were formulated with simplicity, portability, and quality in mind; they maximize

nutrition and help trigger a full effect while minimizing calories. But it's ultimately up to you how you design your meals and
choose your foods, as this book will show in rich detail. Remember, *The Full Diet* is about making sense of all the choices we have
in life today, and learning how to make better choices to support
our weight and fitness goals.

Above all, this is about making your "dieting life" simple
through small, realistic changes that can lead to a lifetime of success and happiness.

The Full Diet is written for anyone who wants to lose weight
and who is not currently morbidly obese. Maybe you've struggled
with your weight for much of your life and you're constantly disappointed by dieting. You may have found some success for short
periods of time. Or perhaps you're among those who have never
found a program that works for you. You've tried a variety of them
without much enthusiasm because they just didn't fit into your
life. *The Full Diet* is also for people who have had surgery and want
to reaffirm their commitment to themselves and tune into where
they are coming from again. This book is not selling surgery. Much
to the contrary, it's dispensing to you the secrets to weight loss
that have been learned (and kept) in the field of obesity surgery.

Remember, if you're morbidly obese, the rules are different.
Morbidly obese people almost always do not benefit from nonoperative weight loss. I do know that some of you reading this may
be interested in bariatric surgery or have had it, and I encourage
you to experiment with the tools and principles I'll be teaching
you here. I've derived much of these strategies from my patients
and what I've learned through their trial and error. Aside from
learning how to properly portion meals or incorporate "cheats"
into your daily eating life, my goals for you include learning how
to be mindful, to be sensible at the table, to pay attention to yourself, and to engage in the real-life eating world with care and self-
respect. You want to say at the end of the day, "I did the best I
could. I'm in control now."

So prepare to make the commitment to never again diet like
you did in the past. I won't tell you to always do something, never

do something, eliminate something from your diet completely, always include something in your diet, or how to behave at every meal. Learn how to do what works for you. By reading my version of a real diet, *The Full Diet*, you'll discover how to:

- End the perpetual obsession with food, eating, dieting, and *work with what's in front of you.* I want to add to your life—not take things away.

- Utilize the *science of fullness*—not appetite—to manage your consumption and satisfy the hunger that resides in the primitive parts of your brain. Appetite is subtle and open to interpretation; full is not so subtle—it's something that everyone can understand.

- Take advantage of the *five intentional steps of digestion* to gain effortless control of your dietary behaviors without resorting to self-discipline or willpower.

- Choose from a variety of practical strategies to achieve sustainable weight loss *regardless of your personal dietary habits and preferences.*

- End the confusion over portion control by *synching visual and physiological cues of fullness.*

- *Be full with less* food but equally as satisfied—if not more so!

- Apply my *cheat prescription* so you can still say yes to indulgences and temptations without feeling that you are losing ground or are a failure.

- Find *fulfillment in a physical activity* that is inexpensive, pleasurable, doable, and convenient.

We live in a world that's hungry for a diet to end all diets. Two out of five women and one out of five men would trade three to five years of their life to achieve their weight goals. Young girls are more afraid of becoming fat than they are of nuclear war, cancer, or losing their parents. Two-thirds of dieters regain weight within a year and virtually all regain it within five years. The failure rates of our country's most popular weight-loss programs exceed 95 percent.

My hope is that *The Full Diet* will lead you to reject the diet mentality that thrives on restrictions, deprivations, self-loathing, and self-defeat, and instead teach you proven principles of fullness that honor your body's innate biology to automatically lose weight without the inner war. This book explores simple changes that can be added to what you *normally* do, based on who you *really* are. When you're full, the core part of your brain where hunger and fullness reside is happy, and it will leave you alone to get on with your life. I want the information in this book to seep into our collective consciousness. The time has come for the diet industry, which banks on failure, to fail itself. Food is not the enemy; traditional diets are.

The Full Quiz:

IS THIS BOOK FOR YOU?

Check as many boxes that you would answer yes to:

☐ Have you ever tried to lose at least ten pounds?

☐ Have you lost at least ten pounds over and over again?

☐ Do you remember the first time you thought about, and became conscious of, your weight?

☐ Have you ever spent $200 on a product or program that you saw on TV (that neither you nor anyone you know had tried or had success with)?

☐ Have you ever drunk vinegar to lose weight?

☐ When you sit down to eat dinner at a restaurant, have you ever thought about avoiding the bread basket?

☐ Do you think a pat of butter is an indulgence?

☐ When you drink a regular Coke or Pepsi, do you wonder if it's killing you?

☐ Have you ever wished you were eating someone else's lunch because it looked so much better than yours?

☐ Have you ever gone to someone else's house and worried about what you're going to eat because they never seem to have something for you?

☐ Have you ever joined a gym thinking you'd go three days a week?

☐ Have you tried to walk 10,000 steps a day using a pedometer?

☐ Have you ever felt guilty about a meal you ate?

☐ Have you ever sneaked a snack or fast food by yourself and hoped "no one would notice or know"?

☐ When you go out with friends for cocktails, do you think about how many calories those drinks will cost your body?

☐ Have you ever negotiated with yourself by saying something like, "If I eat this slice of pizza, I'll have to walk an extra mile tomorrow or skip breakfast"?

☐ Do you think about your weight on a daily basis?

☐ If you were to rank weight loss as a priority in your life, would it be in the top five?

Don't bother counting how many of the above questions you checked. Just a single checked box puts you in the majority. More than one checked box? Still, the majority. Millions of people would answer most of these questions with a resounding *yes*. So you're not alone, and it's time to put an end to all this madness that invades your daily life. Turn the page and let's begin.

PART I

Food Is Not the Enemy; Traditional Diets Are

THE MYTH OF THE GOOD DIETER AND THE TRUTH ABOUT PERMANENT WEIGHT LOSS

Here is how it is supposed to go: You decide that you are unhappy with the way you look and feel. A diet plan or program gets your attention. You buy the book, purchase the plan, or join the program or club. You choose a date to start. You re-create your life to "make this work." This may include throwing out all of your old foods and replacing them with newer, improved, healthier items. You commit to meetings, working out, being "more aware," counting, measuring, weighing, and so on. Then you start. By sheer force of will and determination, you fight to make the plan stick. This is hard when it's all in the face of the many demands and commitments of your real life.

Eventually, the will and force fade. Something always gets in the way. How many people have ever really had long-lasting success in this framework, no matter what support network is established, no matter how many contingency plans are laid out, no matter how much positive reinforcement is given, no matter how good they may be feeling with their small steps toward success?

The discipline flags and the weight comes back—perhaps even more than you started with. You vow to start again soon.

The multibillion-dollar diet industry thrives on your failure. It's built on repeat business—they need you to keep coming back for more. It would be a very short-lived business if we all succeeded the first time. This isn't the only industry that does this. Think about the world of personal printing. Buying a printer is cheap, but keeping it running while constantly putting out ink is expensive. Those ink cartridges will cost you, over and over again as you burn through old ones and buy new ones. The diet and weight-loss industry is similarly structured. You buy into a relatively inexpensive program and then keep going back to it and buying the same—or other—programs and products because the first one didn't result in long-term success. Your original "ink cartridge" isn't going to last a lifetime. The cost of actually carrying out a program and using all of their support material (food, meetings, supplements) is usually a great annuity for the weight-loss companies.

I'm fed up with people trying to lose weight and failing again and again. People are not failing their weight-loss efforts; rather, the industry is failing them. When I ask patients about their weight-loss history, I often hear, "I always go on [name of diet] when I need to lose weight because it works." *Does it?* It sounds like it's failed you every time. Like you, diet programs all insist that they "know how to lose weight." Do they? Do you? If you are holding this book, I'd say not.

The facts of the obesity epidemic are real and significant. So is the fact that we are becoming obsessed with the constant need to control our weight. But our weight obsession is an eternal and fruitless struggle. We are bombarded with facts and scare tactics to make us think we're doomed to die prematurely, never have healthy kids, and be unable to get a good job if we don't lose the extra weight, yet the numbers of obese people are ever increasing. We are more aware, more conscious, yet bigger than ever. We have access to vast resources and options yet we are increasingly failing.

I believe there's a lot to learn from every diet program out there, because virtually all of them have something to teach us. Most are relatively safe and all have their champions—people who have found the diet to work well for them and their life. But another thing they all have in common is this: they ask a lot of you. There's not a diet out there that doesn't ask you to categorically deny or painfully limit some component of what I consider to be a regular, healthy diet with some spontaneity mixed in. I'm not a big believer in forever changing the way you eat just to get your weight-loss goals met. It's just too hard to do. I like to use the rules that you can't avoid, such as how you're wired, and the relationship between your stomach and brain. The more I engage your primitive mind (and you'll soon come to know what I mean by the word *primitive*) and show you success with simple feedback loops, the more you'll believe that my ideas can work for you and the more you'll enjoy the process.

In this chapter, I'm going to begin to shake you loose from the clutches of believing (and returning to the false safe haven) that diets work—that there is the perfect diet out there for you. And I'm going to start by sharing what I reveal to my potential surgical patients during my regular informational seminars.

The perfect diet does not exist. This may seem unbelievable, or just unfair, but diets don't work because they don't take into consideration who we are and what we need. It's a non-negotiable fact.

The Industry Is Built—and Banks—on Failure

It's not too surprising to me that reliable long-term success rates of popular diets are hard to find. How many people who participate in a program by [popular diet X] or [popular diet Y], for example, keep the weight off for good? How many people who go on *The Biggest Loser* sustain their radical transformations? Not many.

> According to a government review, two-thirds of American dieters regain all the weight they lose within a year, and 97 percent gain it all back within five years. Following any of these programs is significantly more expensive than the tried-and-true technique of eating less and exercising more.

A quick wake-up call to the reality behind the "reality" show *The Biggest Loser* merits some attention, because the only realistic element to it may be its stories of failure after the cameras stop recording. The show, as many of you know, achieves rapid transformations worthy of prime-time television drama. Contestants often drop more than 20 pounds in a week through severe calorie restriction and extreme exercise. Add to that some crazy behind-the-scenes dehydration and you've got a recipe for unbelievable weight loss in a short period of time. Ryan Benson won the first season in January 2005 and regained nearly 40 pounds within five days simply by drinking water. Two and a half years after his final weigh-in at 207 pounds, he admitted to reverting back to old habits and weighed almost 300 pounds again. Matt Hoover, the second season's winner, put nearly 15.5 pounds back on within a day of taking home the $250,000 grand prize.

Other contestants who came close to winning tell stories of the drastic measures they took to drop weight fast, such as sitting in a sauna for hours, consuming sugar-free Jell-O for days, and downing diuretic foods to spur water loss. These weight-loss stories may be real, but they certainly are not realistic by any stretch of the imagination, if you consider the means by which they lost weight and the fact that they cannot maintain the loss. The majority of their weight loss came from extraordinary physical activity (four or more hours a day; who has time for that?) and unhealthy dehydration that's unquestionably abnormal. It concerns me that viewers at home start to feel like the proverbial "biggest losers" because they themselves cannot get the miraculous weight-loss results that the contestants experience. Here we go again: you feel like you cannot succeed at yet another diet plan.

Harsh programs like that espoused by *The Biggest Loser* aside, the efficacy of more "normal" commercial weight-loss programs has rarely been evaluated in rigorous long-term trials. You'd think that creators of these programs, which do take an enormous amount of money and research to develop, would want to have this kind of information, especially if it proved that their program worked. That way, they could flaunt their "great results," stomp on the competition, and attract more customers. Something tells me that the statistics—whatever they are for each program—are not that impressive. The success rate of voluntary weight-loss efforts among my patients is, at best, 5 percent over five years.

We do have one scientific report to consider, which was published in the *Journal of the American Medical Association* back in 2003. The researchers compared weight-loss and health benefits, achieved and maintained through self-help weight loss versus with Weight Watchers, the largest provider of commercial weight-loss services in the United States. They looked at both overweight and obese men and women across a two-year period. About half of the participants were sent to Weight Watchers, where they were given a food plan, an activity plan, and lessons during weekly meetings to help them change their eating behaviors. The other half received two 20-minute counseling sessions with a nutritionist and leads on a bunch of self-help resources that they could then access for their information and personal "self-help." Which group did better?

After two years, a total of 150 participants (71 percent) in the commercial group (the Weight Watchers group) and 159 (75 percent) in the self-help group had completed the study. Neither group showed gut-busting weight-loss results. Those who went to Weight Watchers lost, on average, 9.5 pounds at the one-year mark whereas the self-help group dropped a little under 3 pounds. At year two, the Weight Watchers group averaged 6.3 pounds lost and the self-help folks lost 0.44 pounds. Interestingly, the self-help group became a mixed bag of attempts to change diet and increase physical activity: 14 reported using weight-loss medications, another 6 tried herbal products, 10 enrolled in some form of a structured commercial program, and 9 mentioned following an alternative diet plan (for example, protein, Atkins, the Zone) at some point during the two-year study. Changes in the participants' blood pressure, lipids, glucose, and insulin levels were in fact related to the weight loss, but researchers added that there wasn't a significant enough difference between the two groups to say that one approach led to better results than the other by year two.

The point I want to make by this study is that at the end of the day, losing barely ten pounds over the course of a full year of serious effort, and then maybe dropping a few more in the second year by spending all the time and money (and mental anguish) on a formal diet program isn't something to write home about—especially if you want to lose more than ten pounds. How can people who are so successful in so many other aspects of their lives—work, parenting, paying their bills, being good citizens and trusted friends—fail so miserably and predictably every time? Does anyone even believe anymore that a "diet" is going to work and fix weight issues? Let's consider another study, one that really shined a light on the diet industry.

Myth: The "Best" Diet

The largest ever controlled study of weight-loss methods was published in 2009 by the *New England Journal of Medicine*. When researchers pitted the most popular diets against one another, they discovered that it doesn't matter which diet you go on so long as total calories consumed is lessened. More than 800 overweight adults in Boston and Baton Rouge were assigned to one of four diets that reduced calories through different combinations of fat, carbohydrates, and protein. Each plan cut about 750 calories from a participant's normal diet, but no one ate fewer than 1,200 calories a day. Although the diets were not named, the eating plans mimicked those of today's most popular do-it-yourself programs, such as Atkins (low carb), Dean Ornish (low fat), and the Mediterranean diet (low animal protein). Everyone received group or individual counseling during the diet phase.

All of the dieters started to regain weight one year later. I should add that their weight loss during the first year wasn't stunning. At six months, participants in each type of diet had lost an average of 13.2 pounds, and at two years had maintained about 9 pounds of weight loss and a two-inch drop in waist size. After two years, every diet group had lost and regained about the same amount of weight regardless of what diet had been assigned. While the average weight loss was modest, about 15 percent of dieters lost more than 10 percent of their weight by the end of the study. After about a year many participants returned to at least some of their usual eating habits; but they reported an equal level of satiety, hunger, and diet satisfaction.

It does not matter if you are counting carbohydrates, protein, or fat. All that matters is that you are counting something and that your total caloric intake is reduced. You probably cannot live with any of these methods long term, so you need to find a simple, livable approach. I love this study because it finally put to rest the eternal argument between the camps of "who has the best diet." There is no best diet. The only thing that matters is that you DO SOMETHING! The fat versus carbs versus protein craziness is just that—craziness. Sure, there are basic components of your diet to help with energy, proper functioning, and essential nutritional needs. But, aside from having some wise variety in your meals, you do not have to become married to one style of food balance. If you hate diets that emphasize proteins and fat, you are not screwed because "only [name of diet] works."

The real take-home message in this study is that it's necessary to reduce calories. In an insightful editorial, Vanderbilt University's Martin Katahn, Ph.D., puts the study into perspective. He observed that the lower calorie intake was not sustained; all of the subjects lost weight initially but then began to trend back upward at two years. In addition, Dr. Katahn teased out another important fact: there were subjects within each group who did better with weight loss. He noted that these individuals attended more counseling sessions and followed the prescribed dietary changes more closely. He acknowledged that willpower is limited, but he also recognized that the only hope we have of solving the obesity epidemic will be by changing the "environment" that helps us be overweight. I couldn't agree more.

When people ask me why we have such an obesity epidemic today as compared to just a few decades ago, it's clear that genetics play a big hand in loading the gun. And then the combination of environment and our ingrained behaviors pulls the trigger. This second part of the equation—our environment and behavior—encompasses our vulnerabilities, including family upbringing and psychological factors, such as using food for comfort and to manage stress.

Our relationship with food has shifted radically in our lifetime. We've gone from a society where food is primarily all natural and homegrown or handpicked in the farms to one where food is mass-produced, processed, and cheap. The economics of food are sadly structured such that healthy foods cost more and calorie-dense processed and fast foods cost less. In many neighborhoods across the country, it's much easier and cheaper to find a quick burger and fries than it is to buy fresh produce and a lean source of protein that hasn't been genetically altered and chemically enhanced to look better and have a longer shelf life. According to a study headed by UCLA's Center for Health Policy Research, the number of fast-food joints in one's neighborhood has a direct, measurable effect on one's chances of developing diabetes. Case in point: South L.A. has the highest percentage of fast-food restaurants in the city, which has resulted in an obesity rate that is nearly 30 percent of the local population, almost 10 percent higher than the obesity rate in the rest of Los Angeles County.

Among children, the obesity rate is 29 percent, almost 6 percent higher than in the rest of the county.

I could go on and on about the problems with our food supplies and access to healthy, wholesome, weight-friendly meals, but that's not the point of this book. Instead, I'm going to focus on three secrets I've learned through my practice that are supported by the *New England Journal of Medicine* study. The study reveals—and reinforces what I've been saying all along in my practice—that it comes down to three simple things: (1) limiting caloric intake, (2) doing a program that you can sustain, that you believe in, and that fits with what you "like," and (3) changing the "culture" or world that you live in—allowing yourself to create an environment that breeds success in you! And that, my friends, is the whole focus of this book.

The Groundwork: Take an Oath of Weight-Loss Responsibility

I don't operate on everyone who walks through my door seeking help. Prospective patients must undergo a rigorous exam that includes more than a nod to their psychological well-being. Will this person live up to the changes that will inevitably happen in his or her life after surgery? Will she follow my instructions and take my advice seriously long after she is wheeled out of the operating room? Is he prepared for the challenges he will face when he returns to his day-to-day life—with all its temptations, sources of stress, and oversized restaurant portions? Do they know how their physical transformations will ultimately affect their relationships, including with themselves?

Even someone who doesn't use surgery to kick-start weight loss and who makes the changes necessary to shed weight for good has to get past psychological hurdles both during the weight-loss process and afterward. Many of these hurdles are not unlike the ones my patients have to encounter. There's a chronic soliloquy that goes on in most dieters' heads as they contemplate the how, what, where, and why of weight loss. Some of the self-talk that goes on is helpful to the process, but a great deal of it is not—and can actually sabotage any effort to lose weight permanently. This is why it's beneficial to learn what will, versus what will not, help you to meet your goals. After all, why should you waste your mental and physical energy focusing on a lost cause? Let me reveal what those hurdles and self-defeating sermons are. This will enable you to take an oath of weight-loss responsibility.

Give Up Trying to Understand Weight Loss

Before I perform surgery, which involves a significant anatomical rearrangement, I ask my patients to label a diagram to see if they have some idea of what's about to happen (of course, this follows much instruction in previous visits and classes to prepare for surgery). Usually people don't get a perfect score, but they don't have to be too worried about it. I'm the one who needs to know what to do. In my experience, people try to understand too much, especially given the overabundance of information that makes the weight-loss endeavor all the more complicated, confusing, and challenging. I would no more expect you to understand how to do your own gastric bypass than I would have you understand the intricacies and subtleties of weight control. The science of it is staggering and ever-changing. What's more, everyone's personal physiology is different; what may work for your sister might not work for you.

I know that most of you, if not all of you, have read every glossy magazine article on weight loss. Like my patients before surgery, you've attended a number of classes, support groups, and information meetings on just this subject. Statistically, you've read no fewer than eight books on weight loss and fitness. If you spent as much time and effort on researching anything else, you'd be considered somewhat of an expert! You have seen so many repackaged generic messages about protein loading, 30-minute-a-day workouts, tightening your buns, squeezing your butt as you sit in traffic, halving your meals at restaurants, adding grapefruit to your lunches, and so on. You know a lot, right?

The reality is that you know a lot of theory and you know a lot of "stuff to do." Yet you seem unable to incorporate these lessons into your real life. That is the hard part. The painful truth is that you have to put forth the effort to succeed. You have to set yourself up for success—to change what you can stick to. When this doesn't work, then I'll ask you to try other tools. Remember, the only thing that is important is that you actively do something. So stop trying to master the art of weight-loss biodynamics and just focus on doing one thing differently this week. That's where my tools come in. They are designed to help you gain control based on what you're already doing in your everyday life.

As an aside, if you're among the millions who are trying to lose "those last ten pounds" and have been trying to do so for as long as you can remember, you'll find a solution in the next chapter, and it will be an unexpected one. To put it bluntly, if being ten pounds heavier than you want to be makes you feel like a failure, that's really overstating the value of weight in your life.

"Good Dieters" Don't Exist: The National Weight Control Registry, which tracks the habits of some 5,000 successful maintainers, cites a study showing only a fifth of dieters with a history of obesity sustain a loss of 10 percent of their body weight for a year or more. It takes more than following a diet to transform how we live and what we do than deciding to change. Most diets involve a complete transformation on how we encounter food. I think that's asking too much of us. As I spelled out in the introduction, there are very few times in our life when we can make an overnight change and have success. Those times often involve commitments we plan for in advance, such as getting married or choosing to have children. Let's face it: Our time and energy are limited. If the choice is between being there for your work and family and being a good dieter, well, there is no choice. The weight-loss efforts will always lose. They always have.

My patients remember the exact moment when they were conscious of their weight. Did someone say something mean in junior high? Was it when those trendy jeans no longer fit? Was it being way too out of breath after climbing two flights of stairs?

Was it seething after your mom said something? They all vividly recall when they first believed that they were obese. And they all admit that they have never been the same since. When I ask them to remember a time when they didn't think about their weight at all, a look of bliss washes over their face. This isn't special to them, though. I don't know anyone who doesn't believe a life without weight on the brain would be heavenly. I remember going to Boy's Town clothing store to get some new pants before fifth grade started. After unsuccessfully fitting into any pants, the salesman told my mom that I should go over to the "husky" section. I looked him in the eye and said, "I know what that means. You think I'm fat." I do not know who was more shocked—the salesman or my mom. It was my moment that forced me to reflect on who I ultimately wanted to become.

Start with a Vision—for YOU—Not Your Weight

Who do you want to become? Why do you want to become this person? I know this sounds simplistic, but it will be one of your secrets to success. The only way you can mess this up is by believing that the goal has to be grandiose or that you are not qualified to make the change.

As I mentioned previously, a few life-transforming commitments define us and dictate how we interact with the world. In creating a realistic vision for yourself and your weight-loss goals, it helps to consider the following questions in other areas of your life:

- When you got married or committed to a serious, monogamous relationship, how did you then interact differently with those you met? Were you no longer "available," and did you devote most of your personal intimacy energy to the other person in your life? Imagine how miserably you'd fail in the relationship if this were not the case. You've chosen to be in a relationship and all of your other relationships need to fall into place as well.

- If you're a parent, don't you choose to put most of your children's needs before your own? How has your use of time changed since having kids? Are you no longer reckless with safety or casual with your organization? How would a child grow up in a world of impulsivity and chaos? Since becoming a parent, have you changed how you live your life and interact with the world? Are decisions of time and commitment filtered through a sieve of parental responsibilities?

- In your job, have you chosen to pursue a certain line of work or employment with a passion? Even if it is not your dream scenario yet, does it require the dedication of most of your productive waking hours? How does your work define you and your lifestyle? Does it affect your sleep schedule; if, where, and when you drive; how you dress; how you communicate; the way you carry yourself through the day; your e-mail/text/phone obligations; and your overall habits? And does your work influence how you interact with the people you meet?

So you see, we already spend a lot of time working to make ourselves into the person we have decided to be—albeit through our relationships and our professional industry. Anything that we choose to do successfully is a part of a personal transformation, and controlling our weight is no different.

Before you can make any committed effort to take control of your weight, you must start with a vision you have for yourself. In addition to asking yourself who you want to become, it helps to further flesh out your response by asking the following questions:

- How will your weight loss change how you interact with other people and the world at large?

- How will a commitment to losing weight change how you spend your time and energy?

- How will losing the excess weight change your current lifestyle?

- How different is the person you want to become from the person you are now? How so? What other attributes besides your weight do you hope to change in the process?

- Why do you want to become this person? How will the future be different for you?

Don't panic if you cannot answer all of these questions just yet. But you will eventually be able to set clear commitments—and boundaries—with which to pursue your weight-loss goals. You'll also come to know how this process will change your mindset and overall way of life.

Make the Decision

In seventh and eighth grade, I had one friend, Scott. Terminally uncool, we did everything together. During the summer of my eighth-grade year, I learned that Scott was moving away. So I decided that I needed to change everything. I applied to a new school for ninth grade, where I knew no one. I was determined to be "cool," or at least my own '70s version of it. I decided to part my hair in the middle, a trick that took a whole summer to learn and force from my follicles. I dropped the multi-zippered, camp-style shorts in all the colors of the rainbow. I invested in velour shirts. And I decided that I was now an athletic person; I was going to always be on a sports team. When I started at the new school, I said hello to girls instead of avoiding them. I joined the cross-country team. I sat in the quadrangle where the popular people congregated. I acted like I belonged there. And, amazingly enough, I was accepted. I "grew into the role" of being a "cool" kid. I chose not to be so scared of everything, as Scott and I had previously been. I changed my fate.

Fast-forward to after my kids were born. I was a young surgeon in Virginia, fresh out of residency. I had an infant and a two-year-old with a lovely wife who was taxed by her motherly duties. I was trying to study for my board certification, establish a minimally invasive surgery program in southwest Virginia, attempt to do my parental part with my young family, and be a good surgical partner in a very busy multi-specialty practice.

Adding to the load was the fact that I was pretty overweight—by about 50 pounds. To my horror, while playing with the kids and parents in the neighborhood one day, it dawned on me that I was "the fat dad"! How did that happen? The supreme injustice was that this all came on the heels of recent hair loss, too. So, there I was—a bald, fat, responsible dad and surgeon.

When a friend of mine suggested that we "get in shape," I took it to heart, secretly aghast at the idea that my need to get in shape was now a topic of discussion. I decided to confirm the covert messages I was receiving. I immediately looked for proof that I was in fact overweight. I had my wife photograph me in only my shorts so I could see my true "before" self. She summed it up well when she hinted, somewhat delicately, that I looked "like a buffalo." I know she didn't mean it as brutally as it sounded, but there I was—now a bald, fat, responsible, dad, surgeon . . . shaped like a buffalo!

Clearly something had to change. My friend announced that he was going to go to the gym every day before work. I was stunned that he'd indulge his need to "get in shape" by rising at 4:30 in the morning and give up his precious sleep and family time. It seemed like a recipe for being tired, dangerous in the operating room, and neglectful of his family.

But then I realized that I was jealous of him. I wanted to be that guy who made his health and fitness a priority. Soon after his regimen commenced, I watched him skip into work after his morning workout and be all the better because of his exercise. He started bringing his meals to work and missed out on the usual Virginia hospital fare of biscuits and gravy. He filled out his scrubs differently and talked about "feeling so much better." It didn't take long for me to get the hint. This guy was on to something, and I wanted in. I told my wife that I was going to meet my friend every weekday at the gym at 5 A.M. Every day. No exceptions unless I was called in for an emergency. After three months I planned to evaluate if it was worth it.

I still get up at 4:40 in the morning and am working out by 5 A.M. And it all started in 1998 with the simple decision to be the physically active individual that I had always admired. I didn't make it a goal to look like a guy that could be on the cover of *Men's Health*, but I aimed to harness what my body could do and take control of my health. I did not want to be the fat buffalo dad. Period.

Living up to this decision was not easy. Even now, I have to set a minimum of three alarms to make sure I get up. When I started lifting weights, I truly believed that I had torn my biceps because I could not straighten my arms for three full days without assistance. After trying to relearn how to do squats, I could not sit on the toilet for the rest of the week. But over time I learned. I tried program upon program. I hired trainers. I ran a marathon to celebrate my 40th birthday. This was a huge feat for me, as someone who could not run two miles when I started training. It took eight long, slow months of training to prepare me for the event, and now it's crossed off my bucket list.

So again, I ask you to spend time deciding who you want to be. Be specific. I wanted to be the person who was fit and thus made it a priority. I have not regretted this decision. Ever.

Other questions that may be helpful include: What do you want your body to *do* for you? Do you want to be able to run without feeling sick and maybe one day participate in your community's 10K? Do you want to take your kids on vacation next year that will have you swimming, hiking, and biking in nature? What do you love about your life and hate about it? Support those things that you love and explore how to rid yourself of the things that you dislike. Once again, be very specific. If you hate the way you eat impulsively or from stress, we need to think about how to fix that, too. If you are embarrassed or upset by your weight and appearance, then we have to find the tools to fix that, too. If you feel lazy, then we need to address that. You *can* and *should* be the fit, healthy person that you aspire to be so you can participate in life to its fullest. All it takes is first deciding who you want to be and then finding ways to incorporate the tools toward reaching this important goal. I watched life, and then I participated in life. I can unequivocally say that participating is much better.

Find a Role Model

It helps to find a role model as you begin to redefine yourself. Just like I found a role model in my friend at work, you should find someone close to you that can fulfill this role (even if he or she doesn't know it). He may be the person in your office or school who always has time for a workout. You know the type—"I'd love to go to lunch, but that is when I go for my walk." Or the person who lunches at work with food from home and never ventures into the horrific world of fast food. She may say that it's to "save money" or "use up the leftovers"—but I'd bet that she has found the discipline to take control of her meals. Or, maybe they are the people who dare to change their order every darn time they sit in a restaurant to account for their dietary needs. I live with one of them! "No butter, dressing on the side, what can I sub for the white rice, and can I get it broiled instead of fried?"

Stop Hating Yourself

Almost everyone who is unhappy with his or her weight is dissatisfied, frustrated, and oppressed by the constant thoughts about weight. The reasons are many, but they all come down to the fact that weight issues are very public. If you have high blood pressure, people don't look at you and think, *Oh my goodness, she has a very high vascular tone! How could she do that to herself?* If you have diabetes, people don't glare at you and think, *What did he do to his pancreas?* Most health and physical issues are as private as you want them to be. But weight is in a category by itself. It's a billboard advertisement of perceived failures.

The other cruel truth is that it's never just about the weight. The weight becomes a reflection of all one's shortcomings. From all of our weight preoccupation, we become experts at hating ourselves. How many times have you literally hated yourself for your weight? When you think of all that you are and all of the good that you do, and all of the responsibility that you carry on a daily basis—paying the bills, feeding and caring for a family, holding down a job, being nice to others, loving your friends and family—doesn't it seem a tad ridiculous to hate yourself for your weight? Sure, it's convenient. But does it really define you?

When you hate yourself, you subvert any chance of finding out who you really are and your real potential. It becomes all about "losing the weight." And if and when that doesn't play out perfectly, you are intolerant of yourself in the struggle. When does this type of reasoning ever work out? I know of no parent who made a mistake and then was an awful parent forever. The pain of a parental mistake is big. But you have to forgive yourself and move on. You are not the "bad parent" forever. You give yourself a break and you move on. When my son was six months old while I was a trauma resident, I changed his diaper and, in a sleep-deprived stupor, left him next to the sink for a full minute, totally unattended. I forgot to put him back to bed. He was fine and slept through the event, but I wanted to turn myself in to Child Welfare. But I forgave myself (and my wife has almost forgiven me). I learned from the experience and moved on.

For whatever reason, we don't forgive ourselves easily when it comes to our weight. We define ourselves as fat, undisciplined, and failures at dieting. The problem with this is that you lose sight of yourself. The weight is a small part of you. I have to reiterate this again: It's not how you are defined. Let me illustrate this with an example from the world of medicine. When people are diagnosed with cancer, they can become one of two types of patients. There are those who "become the cancer" and define themselves as a walking and talking form of the disease. These people lose hope early on and their prognosis is usually poor. The others see themselves as "people with cancer." They see themselves as separate from the cancer and just have this "thing to deal with" while they get on with their lives. The major attribute that the second group has is that they keep focused on who they are and the realities of how complex and multifaceted they are as humans. They are not just this "one thing." And they maintain hope. They allow themselves to heal, and their prognosis may be much better for it.

When you punish yourself with your negative self-image or by reminding yourself of how much you have failed in weight loss, just stop. No one has the right to think of you that way. No one—not even you! Instead, find out what your real motivations are. It is never as simple as "lose weight." If you really think about it, it is always about a means to an end. Focus on the health aspects of your pursuits. Stop seeing it as being all about what is "wrong" with you. Rather, focus on what you would like to do and how you would like to live. As easy as it is to constantly crap on yourself and your lack of weight-loss success, negative self-talk has never proven to be helpful as a lifelong motivator. The only drivers that work are those that come from creating a reality that you want to live.

If you work to create control in your life . . .

If you stop and consider how good you are "at everything else" . . .

If you look toward creating positive things in your world—health, energy, confidence . . .

Then, you have a fighting chance at making my weight-loss tools work for you.

The Full Challenge: Day 1

Create a vision for yourself that outlines what you want to become within one year. Write out that vision somewhere—a journal, a file in your computer—so you can revisit it often. Explain in as much rich detail as possible how you see yourself one year from now. Avoid using words like *skinny* and *thin,* and instead, focus on larger, more profound goals such as "satisfied with my weight," and "at my goal for cholesterol and blood pressure." Be as specific as you can, and don't limit yourself to just health-related milestones. Think about who you want to become as an individual in terms of your professional and personal goals. How do you want the relationships you maintain to change? How do you want the people you love (i.e., family members, friends, etc.) to see you? You can even include spiritual goals—the things you want to accomplish on a deeply personal level to become a better, more fulfilled you. Perhaps you want to make it a goal of ending your tendency to procrastinate or of working fewer hours over the weekend so you can spend time with family. Whatever it is, make sure it's realistic. If you didn't already answer the questions I posed on pages 15–16, then go back and write out your responses now.

ALLISON CRANDALL

Age: 26, Height: 5'5"
Starting: Weight: 189.4, Size: 15
Final: Weight: 157, Size: 9
Total Lost: 32.4 pounds and 28.25"

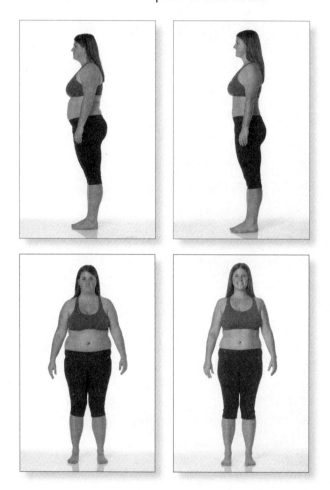

"I'm so much lighter and energetic! I am getting a lot more accomplished on the weekends since I am naturally waking up earlier. I actually sleep through the whole night and feel so well rested in the morning. I've been full since day one and haven't even had a headache from cutting out soda or coffee. Also, I haven't had any cravings, which has made it easy to stick to the plan. I don't know what it is, but out of all the diets I've tried, this has been the easiest."

THERE IS NO NORMAL;
THERE IS ONLY HEALTHY

How much should you weigh?

The media likes to tell us what we should and shouldn't do, and how much we should and shouldn't weigh. But if there's one thing my profession has taught me is that there is no absolute answer to the question of "ideal weight" given a certain set of standards like height, body type, age, and so on.

In this chapter, I'm going to help you set up some parameters for your weight loss. This will entail understanding what it means to be morbidly obese, what an extra 20 pounds can do to the body's physiology, and how you can find a sane weight range. I don't want you to be the chronic dieter looking to lose those last ten pounds, or think you need to lose another ten pounds to be happy. I want you to discover what "healthy" means to you and pursue that health with a passion every day, no matter what you read on the scale.

Lessons from the World of Obesity

Contrary to popular belief, my patients are not the ultimate failures in weight loss. In fact, they are the ultimate success stories for many reasons. First, they are realists. They know that the world of weight-loss programs and diets has nothing for them. They have tried to pee out the pounds by going on liquid diets, or taxed their kidneys by loading up on high-protein, low-carb meals. They have cabbage-souped themselves crazy and parked themselves momentarily on South Beach. They have busted sugar out of their lives in oh-so-many ways. Their inability to lose weight is not from a lack of effort. Rather, they know hundreds who eat the same as they do (or worse) and exercise the same as they do (or less) and manage to have minimal or no weight issues. They know they need something else, and they come to me for help in getting that first tool in the form of a gastric band, sleeve, or bypass. Like any tool, it is only as effective as the person using it. But it gets them started and literally resets their wiring so they are just like the rest of the population. Then I help them find and utilize other post-surgery tools to keep them on track.

No matter how much a person has to lose, the same principles apply to everyone. There are only four reasons to lose weight:

1. To improve your BMI (body mass index, a measure of weight and health).

2. To decrease current medical problems that may be related to weight, such as high blood pressure, diabetes, and so on.

3. To decrease your risk factors for a slew of future health challenges.

4. To prevent weight from messing with your life.

By "messing with your life," I am referring to the persistent and exhausting chatter about weight and its related issues that plague people's subconscious and conscious minds. You know this is true: You're constantly engaged in a recurring thought process about weight. Every meal is an attack. Every snack is a failure. Every indulgence is a weakness. It's not fair to treat yourself so cruelly. Why are you so intolerant of the fact that you have to eat to live? There's a great variety of foods that you can consume to sustain your life. Dieting shouldn't be a constant part of our everyday lives that undermines who we are and what we feel comfortable doing.

Consider the typical experience at a café. Let's say you order a latte and a pastry. Do you simultaneously deal with the mental baggage of wondering whether or not you've made the right choice in milk, sweetener, and cup size for your weight? If the extra 60 calories and 8 grams of fat in the whipped cream that you add is what you really want, then when you say no to this option, don't you feel superior? Do you really think the 100 fewer calories in the low-fat blueberry coffee cake defines who you are any better than the regular coffee cake? And when you choose the sugar-free pastry, do you feel like you've accomplished something? What about the additional fat the manufacturer has probably added by not using sugar?

These examples just touch the surface of the kind of madness that millions of people go through on a daily basis. I'm going to show you how to end this chaos and let you define the foods in your life, including the treats, so that they won't wreak havoc on your psyche or make you want to give up.

Even though you may initially aim to reduce the severity of medical conditions related to your weight, such as high blood pressure and cholesterol, if you focus on just one reason alone, all the other reasons will be addressed, too. In other words, you'll not only help treat your current medical conditions, but you'll also decrease your BMI, risk for other health challenges, and you'll feel better about your weight and its real role in your life.

All reasons to lose weight boil down to these three things: *fear, need,* and *desire.* (Desire should be a distant third to fear and need.) We fear what excess will do to us physically and emotionally; we need to feel in control of our weight, and we strongly desire to be happy with our weight. If the topic of weight loss weren't so pervasive, then these statistics wouldn't be so astonishing:

- More than one out of three "normal dieters" progress to pathological dieting, which means just as it sounds: a disordered behavior characterized by chronic dieting. One-fourth of those who diet endlessly will suffer from partial- or full-syndrome eating disorders. And we're not just talking about anorexia nervosa and bulimia. At the other end of the spectrum, an eating disorder can entail gorging on food or just *thinking* about food and weight to the point that those thoughts are intrusive and oppressive to daily life.

- Almost half of American children between first and third grades say they want to be thinner.

- Four out of five ten-year-old children are afraid of being fat.

- Half of our nine- and ten-year-old girls say that being on a diet makes them feel better about themselves.

- About 25 percent of American men and 45 percent of American women are on a diet on any given day.

Clearly, the problem isn't just tormenting our adult society, but it's also changing the way our children think as they try to mature into thoughtful, self-loving, independent adults.

You Get to Define Healthy

I'm not the type of doctor who likes to impose numbers and formulas on my patients. I'm the anticalorie counter and antidiet programmer. But in my world, I do have to respect some of the basic tenets of measuring health, such as BMI and what it means, to understand from a scientific standpoint what it means to be "overweight." Using a formula to calculate obesity is not a new concept. In the 19th century, a Belgian statistician named Adolphe Quetelet came up with the Quetelet index of obesity, which measured obesity by dividing a person's weight (in kilograms) by the square of his or her height (in inches). Before 1980, doctors generally used weight-for-height tables—one for men and one for women—that included a range of body weights for each inch of height. These tables were limited because they were based on weight alone, rather than body composition.

Body mass index (BMI) is defined as the individual's body weight divided by the square of his or her height, commonly seen as kg/m^2. BMI can also be determined using a BMI chart (see the box on page 28 for a cheat sheet of BMI values). BMI became an international standard for obesity measurement in the 1980s, and the public got wind of it in the late 1990s when the government launched an initiative to encourage healthy eating and exercise.

The current BMI chart is not as exact a science as you might think or have been led to believe. In 1998, the National Institutes of Health lowered the overweight threshold for BMI from 27.8 to 25 to match international guidelines. The move added 30 million Americans who were previously in the "healthy weight" category to the "overweight" category. What's more, this method of measurement can be skewed for people who carry a lot of (heavy) muscle mass or, conversely, who lack lean muscle tissue but have high body fat despite low overall weight. BMI categories do not take into account many factors such as frame size and muscularity. The categories also fail to account for varying proportions of fat, bone, cartilage, water weight, and more. Using BMI for athletes, for example, can overestimate their level of body fat because muscle is denser than fat and weighs more. An athlete's body fat can be normal or even low, but the person may have a high BMI. This does not mean that they are unhealthy or overweight. A number of gold medal–winning athletes at the Olympics would be considered obese based solely on their BMI. Similarly, taller people may have a BMI that is uncharacteristically high compared to their actual body fat levels due to how BMI is calculated.

Use the BMI chart in Appendix A (page 203) to pinpoint a general range for yourself in pounds. This chart is just a guide and may not apply to everyone. You may not fall exactly into your "normal" range given your height. This chart does not factor body composition into the equation, so it does not take into account different body frames and build, muscle mass and tone, and so on.

Body Mass Index Table

BMI (Body mass index) = Weight in kg/(height in meters)^2

Category	BMI
Underweight	< 18.5
Healthy weight	18.5–24
Overweight	25–29
Obese	30–34
Severely overweight	35–39
Morbidly obese	40–49
Super obese	50–60
Ultra obese	> 60

Based on BMI numbers across the American population, 64 percent of adults are overweight and 32 percent of children are overweight. Thirty-four percent of adults over the age of 20 are considered obese and 16 percent of children are obese.

Should you know your BMI and use it to measure your progress down the weight-loss path? Or should you go by the scale? Or how your clothes fit?

These are all good questions. You'll find their answers on your own. It helps to have some sort of a baseline from which to measure your progress, and I think we all tend to become attached to certain barometers that clue us into whether or not we are moving forward or need to adjust course. But we also have to be careful how seriously we regard those barometers and how much our emotions become wrapped up in what they reveal. A woman who is 5'4" would have to weigh 145 pounds to have a healthy BMI of 25. Yet many women who are 5'4" think this is too heavy for them.

I can't honestly tell you what your ideal weight is. In my opinion, an appropriate weight is one where you: (1) feel healthy,

(2) are living the life you want to live (that is, you are participating in life and thoughts about weight are not dragging you down), and (3) you feel comfortable in your skin. Can you achieve these three goals? Absolutely. For this reason, I recommend that you focus less on your BMI or finding a specific number on the scale, and instead, accept a weight *range*. The following chart shows weight and BMI ranges based on height. This is simply a guide to help you identify a range. You may not know your actual range until you reach it and allow yourself to be happy there. My guess is that when you reach that range, you will also have reached a healthy BMI, too.

I understand that this advice is counter to what other experts, or even your doctor, might say. I also understand that you may feel frustrated by not having "a number" to fixate on and put all of your efforts toward reaching. But I want you to approach this weight-loss process with an entirely new perspective. Your past efforts to reach a size X or a weight Y have not worked. So bear with me. Try to evict your rigid rules and straitlaced objectives from your mind. Instead, embrace a different modus operandi. This could be the secret to your forthcoming lasting success.

A Little Weight Goes a Long Way

Though we all are aware that obesity is a big problem today, affecting about 25 percent of the industrialized world, it would be neglectful of me to skip over the recent observations and studies in this area, some of which are surprising and can be sources of motivation.

In America today, more than a third of the adult population is now obese (defined as having a BMI of more than 30). The cultural meaning of obesity has changed at the same time. For much of human history, fatness has been a sign of prosperity, of having climbed the social and economic ladder. But now obesity in Western societies is concentrated among the poorest and least educated. Furthermore, there are discrepancies among different ethnicities.

In America, for instance, blacks are 50 percent more likely to be obese than whites, and Hispanics 20 percent more likely.

> The average American is 23 pounds overweight and consumes 250 more calories than was consumed two to three decades ago.

To date, obesity has been linked with more than 30 serious medical conditions. About 400,000 obesity-related deaths occur each year in the United States alone, making it the second-leading preventable cause of death after smoking. And the economics of fat are staggering. According to the Centers for Disease Control and Prevention and RTI International, a nonprofit research institute, obesity-related medical expenses accounted for 9.1 percent of all annual medical costs in 2006, up from 6.5 percent in 1998. Annual health-care costs of obesity in America have risen from $74 billion in 1998 to $147 billion in 2008.

Making matters worse, the health-care costs and lost productivity caused by obesity contribute to American manufacturers relocating to countries where the population hasn't been saddled with this problem. And, interestingly, according to a 2006 study performed by researchers at the University of Illinois at Urbana-Champaign and Virginia Commonwealth University, Americans spent $2.8 billion more on auto gasoline in 2005 than in 1960 due only to the extra body weight in vehicles. This study used data on U.S. weight gain from 1960 to 2002—a period in which the weight of the average American increased by more than 24 pounds—and factored out other variables, such as increased cargo weight or decreased fuel efficiency due to poor maintenance, while accounting for inflation. This is just one example that shows that the costs of obesity go well beyond what we imagine.

In another study that emerged in 2010, researchers from George Washington University determined that obesity costs men an average of more than $2,600 extra each year, and women pay more than $4,800 extra. The disparity between the sexes is due to data showing that obese women earn less than skinnier women.

The most crushing research findings of late have looked at the effects of obesity on our children. Childhood obesity has more than tripled in the past 30 years, with a mind-blowing one-third of America's youth now overweight or obese and almost 10 percent of infants and toddlers dangerously heavy. Doctors are now treating childhood conditions that were previously monopolized by adults: high blood pressure, high cholesterol, and type 2 diabetes. Many children are stigmatized and suffer from low self-esteem, which can lead to depression. If current trends continue, nearly one in three kids born in 2000—and one in two minorities—will develop type 2 diabetes in their lifetime, according to the American Diabetes Association. The disease is linked to heart attack, stroke, blindness, amputation, and kidney disease. A study published in early 2010 found that obese children are more than twice as likely to die prematurely as adults than kids on the lower end of the weight spectrum.

Regardless of age (or race, gender, ethnicity, or religion), smaller weight gains also carry ill health effects. Even a scant 10 or 20 extra pounds increases the risk of disease and death. On the flip side, it takes only a small weight *loss*—as little as 5 percent—to gain great health benefits. For a person who weighs 200 pounds, that is just 10 pounds! Weight loss is vital in the treatment and prevention of heart disease, unhealthy blood cholesterol levels, heart failure, high blood pressure, sleep apnea, gallbladder disease, osteoarthritis, diabetes, and other chronic diseases. In fact, here's a quick summary of just a few of the benefits of losing a modest amount of weight, around 5 to 10 percent of initial body weight:

- Weight loss reduces the risk of breast cancer when the weight is lost before age 45.

- Weight loss decreases blood pressure and reduces risk of heart disease.

- Weight loss increases HDL ("good") cholesterol incrementally.

- Weight loss reduces the incidence of type 2 diabetes by 58 percent.

- Weight loss increases your life expectancy by about seven years.

The latest studies from the National Cancer Institute and other research institutions suggest that more than 20 percent of all cancers are associated with overweight or obesity. For many years, researchers have been telling us that certain forms of cancer that are linked to hormones are due to side effects of being overweight. For example, a government report on overweight and obesity has summarized that obesity increases the risk of breast cancer after menopause because body fat produces the hormone estrogen.

The strongest correlation between weight and illness is found with diabetes. Weight gain significantly increases diabetes risk; more than 80 percent of people with type 2 diabetes are overweight or obese. The risk increases about 25 percent for every unit increase in BMI over 22. One study estimated that more than a quarter of new diabetes cases could be due to a weight gain of 11 pounds or more. If we were to eradicate adult weight gain and obesity, we could eliminate more than 80 percent of all diabetes. It's not surprising that one of the first treatment recommendations for diabetes is weight loss.

I've seen the dramatic effects of weight loss on diabetes firsthand. For many of my patients, the curative effects of weight-loss surgery on their diabetes are extraordinary. Within days of surgery, their diabetes vanishes—even before the weight begins to notably fall off. When I share this with a roomful of prospective patients— many of whom suffer from this chronic and often debilitating condition—the disbelief and amazement are palpable. The thought of living without relying on diabetes medication and the threat of the illness's potential health implications and complications is just unreal. But it's true: studies now show that gastric bypass surgery may prevent or reverse type 2 diabetes, even for patients on the lower end of the obesity scale, and even without any weight loss.

Explaining how this happens requires more than a biochemistry class, and we don't yet have all the answers. We are just beginning to understand how the gut plays a defining role in the sophisticated hormonal system, especially with regard to the regulation of insulin production and sensitivity. When you change the anatomy of the stomach, you change the biochemistry of your body. Last year, 22 international medical and scientific groups backed a consensus statement recommending less stringent weight guidelines for gastric bypass surgery for patients with diabetes. I myself have given talks at the American Diabetes Association to raise awareness as to the profound effects gastric surgery can have on diabetes. More studies are needed, but in a few years it wouldn't surprise me to see the number of surgical candidates increase as evidence of diabetes being a surgically fixable disease accumulates and we bring moderately obese patients with diabetes into the same fold as those who qualify now for the procedure.

Weighing too much can also have unexpected and devastating health repercussions beyond the usual diabetes and heart-health concerns. Recent studies have found that if you are an overweight woman, you may have a harder time getting health insurance or have to pay higher premiums; are at higher risk of being misdiagnosed or receiving inaccurate dosages of drugs; are less likely to find a fertility doctor who will help you get pregnant; and are less likely to have cancer detected early and get effective treatment for it. This is unfortunate news, and fat discrimination is partially to blame. A 2008 Yale study suggested that discrimination against overweight people—particularly women—is as common as racial discrimination. Bias can start when a woman is as little as 13 pounds over her highest healthy weight. Men apparently get more leeway, and are not at serious risk for weight bias until their body mass index reaches 35 or higher. These statistics show that weight has a kind of domino effect for other social ills. Our weight goes a long way in affecting how we are judged and stereotyped in our culture.

What's Really Bothering You?

Weight control is often a great distraction from—or a disguise for—what's really bothering a person. Too often I hear patients state that after the weight is gone, they finally realize that they still have problems. In other words, it wasn't necessarily the weight that impeded their happiness. To this end, I want you to find out what truly motivates you to lose the weight and keep that foremost in your mind as you proceed. It's critical to have a concrete reason that goes far beyond a vague notion of happiness, because weight loss doesn't necessarily yield happiness. This exercise builds on the one you did in the previous chapter when you asked yourself who you want to become and what you want your body to do for you. If you haven't yet answered these important questions, now is the time.

My patients typically are not concerned with fitting into a size 2 pair of jeans. They want to lose weight for more monumental reasons. They want to fit into a seat on a rollercoaster with their friends. They want to play with their kids and grandkids. They want to feel sexy and desired. They want to stop being the "largest person in the room." They don't want to ask for seatbelt extenders on airplanes. They want to be able to fit into clothes at the Gap. They want to put an end to the serious health conditions they have from carrying too much weight. And they don't want their friends and family to worry about them. They are tired of their weight defining them. Your reasons for picking up this book may be similar. Though you may not have nearly as much weight to lose as one of my patients, the end results could likewise change your life for the better.

Let me give you a vivid example. I once treated a woman I'll call Jenny, who had a Lap-Band procedure and who went from weighing 265 pounds down to 145 at 5'4" tall. Her BMI had dropped from 45 (putting her into the "morbidly obese" category) to 25 ("healthy") when she weighed in a year and a half after her surgery. We spoke at length about her experience. Jenny was now a size 8, happily dating again, training for her first sprint triathlon, and thrilled that people were making eye contact, holding doors open for her, and giving her more responsibility at work. In the Costco parking lot, she had an encounter with a man she initially assumed was stalking her, but he was really just interested in finding out who she was and if she was available to date. Jenny felt woefully incapable of dealing with this kind of attention. She spent a full 20 minutes describing to me what her plan was to lose another ten pounds.

Jenny then guiltily began describing the indulgences she'd had at a recent work party, reporting that she found herself eating and drinking "the wrong things" and how it reminded her of her old self. As she crossed and uncrossed her legs, a feat she couldn't do 120 pounds ago, she expressed her real worry about the fact she would never get to her goal weight. I abruptly stopped her diatribe against herself and told her that it was time to change not just how much she wanted to weigh but how she was defining herself. I said, "This may freak you out, but I'm going to tell you to do something that you've never heard before. I'd like you to be happy with your weight now and stop trying to lose more. Your BMI is 25, which is perfect. You look phenomenal. Your life is now amazing. And if you allow yourself to be, you could be totally happy."

Jenny burst into tears and said, "I can't do that. I have no idea what I'm going to do with myself if I'm not unhappy about my weight." I had heard this before from other patients. Since youth, Jenny's life had been defined by her weight. Her mother harassed her as a child due to her weight. She had joined Weight Watchers as a 12-year-old. She could recall her first experience shopping at Lane Bryant for plus-sized clothes, as well as the potential jobs she had lost due to weight discrimination. For as long as Jenny could remember, her life revolved around her weight. She admitted: "That's just who I am—a person who struggles with her weight. I don't think I'm capable of not thinking about it. It feels like a part of every moment in my life."

To that I said, "You've been profoundly damaged, and it's going to take a lot of work to get over the trauma that society has inflicted on you. More important, you've accepted a lot of this abuse as truth and then traumatized yourself over and over again. I'd like to see you back in two weeks, and every time you think that you need to lose more weight, I want you to think about the fact that Dr. Snyder disagrees with you. All I want you to do is say thank-you to everyone who says you look great. Every time you think you have to lose more weight, you have to say to yourself: 'I am perfect where I am.' And, after a few years, you may actually believe it."

How different are you from Jenny? You may not be 120 pounds overweight or at risk for serious illnesses, but if I told you to take an entire day off from thinking about your weight, could you do it? If the answer is no, then you know what I'm going to say: your weight struggles are too important to you. And you're wasting a lot of time, effort, and heart.

Are you thinking about your weight to this degree because it's an easy target on which to focus your anxieties and fears? Does it distract you from your real issues and concerns? Is weight the fall guy in your life? As Jenny so clearly articulated to me that day, she wasn't sure if she could take on the responsibility of *not* having weight as the cause of all the ills in her life. I have had patients gain back a notable amount of weight because it was easier for them to blame the weight than it was to take control of their lives and accept full responsibility. Could this be true for you?

The Full Challenge: Day 2

Your challenge for today is to go through a short series of exercises that sum up the ideas I've presented so far. Be honest. You don't have to share any of this with others. If you choose to write in a journal, which I highly recommend, no one else has to read it. Facing your feelings about your weight and how much it affects your everyday life is an essential step in your journey to living a full life.

Exercise #1

Keep a journal or piece of paper on hand today so you can easily make a note each time you think about your weight. Each time weight enters your mind, jot down the time and record how you're feeling emotionally. This can be any number of things: tired, sad, hungry, lonely, happy, fat, stressed, frustrated, anxious, excited, and so on. Feel free to add any additional notes to describe the source of your emotions. For example, if weight crosses your mind when you feel stressed, you may add something like "stressed: my credit card bill just arrived and I don't think I can pay it this month."

Exercise #2

I ask my patients to list all of the weight-loss efforts they have tried, how long they spent trying to make the plan or diet work, how much weight they lost, how much they regained, and how much money they spent. Virtually everyone has an epic list and adds, "and that's all I can remember," meaning that there are a lot more that they cannot remember or have chosen to forget! Not a recipe for success. So I'm going to ask the same from you. List all the weight-loss efforts or programs you've tried. If you can, add how much you lost on any given program, how much it cost, and how much you regained. It's okay to guesstimate. This isn't a test. It's simply a way for you to actually see the stark reality of your past pursuits so you can embrace a new approach. It will amaze you that you actually remember "losing 18 pounds on Weight Watchers when you were first out of college."

Exercise #3

Vow not to try any of the diets you listed in exercise 2 again. In fact, take an oath to never diet again like you have in the past. Check the following statements as confirmation:

☐ I will give up trying to understand weight loss.

☐ I will keep my weight struggles in perspective relative to other areas of importance in my life.

☐ I will continue to ask myself, "Who do I want to become?" and will live up to that answer every day.

☐ I will seek role models to keep me on track and living up to the vision I have for myself.

☐ I will stop hating myself and defining myself by my weight.

As a doctor, you know that I can make more oblique references to healthy weight. Do you know your heart calcium score? Lipid ratio? Waist circumference? Unless we're talking about life-threatening illness and debilitation, I don't think you need to be engaged in such scholarly pursuits. These questions feed into your masochistic need for me to figuratively beat you up. Stop! Let's just get practical control over things you can actually control. Get a checkup with your general practitioner. Make sure your basic health indexes are in line, and then let's work on moving on with your life. You'll feel like a fat slob if your waist circumference is two inches bigger than it's supposed to be. Do you need that abuse from me? No. You don't need that information to control your weight better. Stop spending so much energy trying to define the problem. Instead, put all your energy into finding a solution that works for you.

No one knows what you are capable or incapable of but you. So why accept a one-size-fits-all approach? To create a private-label program for you, you need to find the tools that will work for you and learn how to fold them effortlessly into your life as you would ingredients into a batter. Some tools will work for you and some will not. Since these tools cost little or nothing, you can always use the "money back guarantee" of abandoning them and trying others.

Exercise #4

Find a comfortable, safe place to sit down where you'll be undisturbed and free to let your mind roam. I'm going to ask a series of questions that I encourage you to think about and respond to in your mind or, preferably, in your journal. Some of these may be difficult to answer right away, and if that's the case, come back to them later once you've let them simmer in your head for a few days. Or write down what you can today and add to them later. Remember, all of what you record is for your eyes only.

- Aside from my weight, where is the tension in my life? List and describe as best you can. (Consider your relationships, home life, financial security, career/job, and health.)

- What do I think my life would be like without weight being an issue and a daily concern? Describe.

- List one way in which losing weight will *enhance* my life.

- List one way in which losing weight will *take away from* my life.

- List all the reasons why I want to lose weight. (List both monumental reasons [for example, controlling or eradicating my diabetes and hypertension] and more superficial ones [that is, feeling more attractive and fitting into my jeans better]. All of these reasons count and can help you stay motivated for permanent change.)

- What do I want my weight loss to do for me? (It's okay if the answers to this question overlap with other responses. It doesn't hurt to reaffirm your reasons.)

- What do I want my *body* to do for me? (Again, you can restate reasons you've already thought about and written down.)

- Aside from weight loss, what do I want to accomplish in my life? List at least five things.

I know it sounds ridiculous, but success at weight loss can be hard to accept, especially if your weight-loss struggles have come to define who you are. What will life be like without a weight problem? If your life is actually relatively good despite your weight challenges, then you also need to think about why you continue to hold onto the need to struggle with weight. Is it because you must have *something* wrong in your life? Does having a pretty perfect life seem unreasonable to you? Really take the time to think about these questions. They may be especially relevant if you're among those who have the "last ten pounds" burned into your mind. If there is no serious tension in your life except for the fact that you're not happy about your weight, you would do well to stop and reflect on this. If you're at a healthy weight, why can't you be happy where you are now?

The constant pursuit of a "goal weight" for many people is such a big part of life that the thought process of extricating themselves from this eternal battle can be a monumental task. When you reach your goal weight, do you believe you'll be able to turn this off as you would switch off a faucet? My concern is that there is no end point for you. It's not about the constant

41

pursuit; it's about establishing a healthy mind-set. I'm thrilled when I see a woman about 10 to 12 pounds from her goal weight and she's happy. You should not tolerate an endless pursuit of weight loss and eternal dissatisfaction with your results. It's a contaminated way of thinking.

Exercise #5 (optional)

Sometimes I tell patients (half jokingly!) to go to their local tattoo parlor and have today's date etched in a small, inconspicuous place on their body. Whenever they are tempted to try another diet, they can look at that tattoo and remember: "This is the day I promised myself not to diet any longer." Alternatively, see if you can find another way to remember this oath. Write today's date in permanent ink on your bathroom wall or in your shower so you can see it every morning. Write out the "This is the day" statement and have it framed so you can hang it in your kitchen or bedroom, or sitting on your desk at work. Find a lucky charm with today's date on it and keep it in your purse or car. You may not want to go to these extremes, but I'm serious about making the commitment to never diet the way you have in the past again. Ever.

ERIC KING

Age: 40, Height: 6'2"
Starting: Weight: 224.6, Size: 38"
Final: Weight: 187, Size: 33"
Total Lost: 37.6 pounds and 26.25"

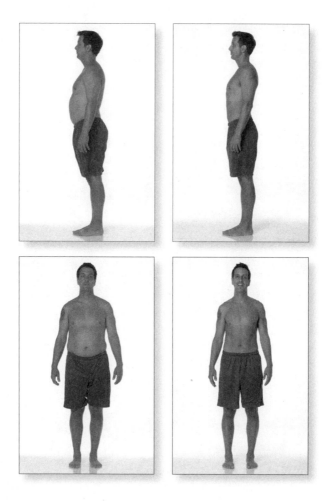

"I've seen so many changes in my body, and everyone else keeps commenting on my 'dramatic weight loss.' My clothes are much looser, and I've moved three belt notches. I follow my own healthy diet and avoid sugar, bread, and alcohol. I live at the beach, so being comfortable with my shirt off is key!"

PART II

The Full
Effect

CHAPTER THREE
DAY 3

THE SCIENCE OF FULLNESS

Most of us have a favorite restaurant where we like to go with friends or family and let our appetites run loose. I commiserate with patients on this experience all the time, talking about how we sit ourselves down, order whatever we want, and pay little attention to cues of fullness until it's far too late. Picture, for example, a night at your favorite steakhouse where you really pack it in—drinks, a loaf or two of bread, artichoke spinach dip, shrimp cocktail, salad with all the trimmings, porterhouse steak smothered in mushrooms, baked potato with all the fixings, and chocolate cake for dessert. (And if steak and potatoes are not your thing, then just substitute whatever place you like to go to and indulge from start to finish.) It's a two-hour affair where reaching for another sip of wine or beer and inhaling copious courses of food happens automatically. Afterward, you hobble to your car feeling bloated and clandestinely undo the top button on your pants so you can breathe easier. Now, at this exact moment, what if I asked you, "Do you want to go for some ice cream?"

You'll look at me like I'm a lunatic. You are FULL! How could you ever think of eating ice cream now? Before you ate the huge meal, ice cream after dinner sounded fantastic. You may have even thought of which flavor you'd get. So why are you in control now? What changed? Well, it's because your primitive, hypothalamic brain has taken over. It trumps any cravings you may have. You are, by every definition of the word, full.

I don't have to expound on what fullness means from the scene I just described. You know what it's like because you've experienced this countless times. Let's turn now to the scientific perspective on fullness, and how the biological cascade of events that takes place brings about that sensation. Along the way you'll also learn how gastric bypass and banding surgery work; and how they apply to understanding your own genetic, physical, and psychosocial make-up. In subsequent chapters, this scientific view will give you the foundation for applying the right weight-loss tools to your life.

Be Full, Not Satisfied

Much is made of the word *satiety* in diet circles, and it's very confusing. Satiety is a concept that is open to interpretation. In the eating world, we can be satisfied and still eat a brownie. Satisfaction allows us to slow down; it does not necessarily make us stop. Habits, emotions, and convenience allow us to violate the limits that our "satisfaction" put on us. But "full" is another story. When we are full, a primal, prehistoric characteristic that exists in all of us takes over. I'll be explaining this shortly. We cannot ignore full. To do so is uncomfortable. Full is not open to interpretation or negotiation.

In my bariatric surgery practice, I am very aware of the science of fullness from all angles—physical, hormonal, emotional, and psychological. When people ask me to explain it all in a few brief sentences, I compare it to the attributes of love, because the more I learn about and investigate fullness as a doctor—and a caretaker of morbidly obese patients—the more I realize that comprehending fullness is a lot like understanding love. We have a pretty good idea of how love affects people physically and hormonally. Signs of love's impact on a person are evident in an increase in heart rate, a narrowing of the pupils, and a warm flush on the skin. These are straightforward and well-defined reactions to the experience of lust or love. But, the *feeling* of love, that is something more complex, a sum of all parts that entails not just the physical and hormonal effects but also the less concrete sensations from our emotions and psyche. I see fullness in the same light. The individual parts that we

48

can trace from a purely scientific standpoint are important, but the sum of all our physical and psychological experiences is what defines the whole essence of fullness. And nowhere does that essence play itself out so clearly as in its survivalist underpinnings that date back to our earliest ancestors.

The Full Effect

Just as each of us is hardwired to feel hungry, every one of us is hardwired to feel full. Our innate circuitry for fullness has been encoded in human genes for millions of years, for longer than we've had drive-thru restaurants, farmers' markets, or the ability to mass-produce food. In fact, the precise biology of this fascinating process involves an effect similar to that in the use of narcotics. But before I get to the details that also compare it to narcotics, let me first describe the process with the help of a car analogy.

Overall, the basic physical journey toward fullness is similar to how a car's fuel system works. When you go to the gas station, you're starting a simple feedback loop. As you fill your car's gas tank, the fuel gauge on the dashboard indicates the tank's level of fullness with the help of a sensor. At some point, the indicator on your dashboard says *F* for *Full*. This prevents you from overfilling the tank and spilling fuel. Now picture your stomach as a tank and your brain as the dashboard fuel gauge—and a very primitive one at that.

We tend to think about keeping our stomachs happy, but we should really be focusing on our brains—our ancient, reptilian brains—because that's where true fullness resides. Contrary to what seems logical, you are not full when your stomach is full; technically, you are full when your primitive brain believes that your stomach is full and tells you that you're full. The obvious next question becomes: how do you get your brain to believe you are full? Of course, it's important to understand the general relationship between your brain and the rest of your body. This is true about everything we experience in our physical lives. When you step on a tack (pin side up), for instance, it's not your foot that actually hurts; it's your *brain* deciding that the impulses from your foot indicate "hurt." People cannot feel this pain if they have

49

nerve or spinal injuries that prevent signals from traveling from foot to brain. They will still injure their foot, but they won't experience the physical pain like the rest of us do. In the case of fullness, that undeniable "full" sensation is felt after your brain—and, more specifically, your hypothalamus—has interpreted all the signals coming in that originate in your stomach, the anatomical organ between your esophagus and small intestine where the real magic begins on both a physical and hormonal level.

If we could cast back to millions of years ago and visit our ancestral cavemen and women, we'd find that the hypothalamus functions exactly the same now as it did then. This is where your inner reptile lives and makes certain demands of you. An exceedingly ancient structure that sits in the middle of your head, the hypothalamus is unlike most other (more sophisticated and advanced) brain regions, and has maintained a striking similarity in structure throughout the course of human evolution. We'd even find remarkable similarities in the hypothalamus of animals that came long before mammals roamed the earth. Evolving around the time of the dinosaurs, this part of the brain serves an important purpose: to beat starvation. In the absence of food, the hypothalamus is responsible for releasing biological chemicals that change how the body functions so it can successfully (and hopefully) find food to survive. For example, when faced with real starvation, the hypothalamus will trigger the secretion of a hormone called *orexia*, which, in tiny doses, can have an overwhelming and profound effect. It will make you acutely more alert, increase your muscle efficiency, and heighten problem solving—all in the name of finding food quickly or risk death.

The hypothalamus does more than simply control hunger and serve as your psychological eating center. It helps to think of it as a special type of command center for your entire body, a headquarters for maintaining the body's preferred status quo, sometimes referred to as its homeostasis or "balance." It houses several important centers that preside over a wide range of physiological functions, including body temperature, thirst, water balance, circadian rhythms (for example, sleep-wake cycles), fatigue, escape from danger, contractions during childbirth, and even arousal and sexual function. We owe many universal experiences, such as pleasure, aggression, stress, embarrassment, and aversion to our hypothalamus, which is fully functional the moment we are born. One of its most important jobs is to link the nervous system to the hormonal system; this is possible through the help of the pituitary gland, a pea-sized structure that dangles off the bottom of the hypothalamus and which actually secretes those behavior-altering hormones as dictated by the hypothalamus. Although the pituitary usually steals all the credit for being the master hormonal gland, in reality it's the consummate servant to the hypothalamus.

Speaking of hormones, a lot has been written about ghrelin and leptin in recent years, the two appetite hormones that play a supportive role in our feelings of hunger and fullness. I'll get to the hormonal reactions in the body's quest for fullness shortly. But first, we must cover the gateway to fullness that's largely absent from discussions about hunger and appetite. At one end of the fullness spectrum we have the hypothalamus, and at the other—the genesis of fullness—we have another unique region in the body.

The Heart of the Matter: The Cardia: Few people (except maybe we bariatric surgeons who work with the physical anatomy of fullness on a daily basis) realize that the heart, quite literally, triggers fullness in the top 10 percent of the stomach. To discredit the anatomy of fullness and concentrate just on the related hormonal reactions to eating is like missing the forest for the trees. Let me explain.

There's a reason the top 10 percent of your stomach is called the "cardia" in gastric medicine circles. Located near your heart, it's where a legion of stretch receptors reacts to food physically filling your stomach. Recall how I explained that the hypothalamus connects your nervous system with the omnipotent hormonal system to influence your behavior (that is, whether you drink a glass of water to quench thirst, run for your life to escape a burning building, or stop at a fast-food joint to cater to your hunger). In terms of eating, as your hamburger and French fries mechanically stretch out your cardia, a series of events follows, starting with a special nerve called the vagus nerve, which communicates with your hypothalamus that you're filling up. Biology aside, it makes sense that we

51

should have a built-in way to prevent food from moving upstream and overflowing into our esophagus, which would be extremely uncomfortable not to mention gross. But those stretch receptors in the upper stomach can only tell part of the story. As with other indicators in the body, they need help in relaying the message to the brain in order to complete the story, and the sensation of fullness.

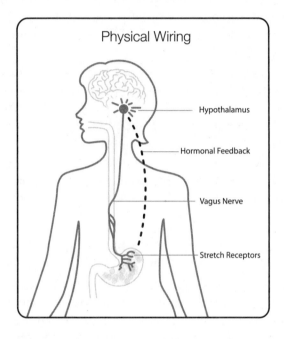

The vagus nerve (which literally means "wandering nerve") is the longest of the cranial nerves; it wanders from the brain stem through organs in the neck, chest cavity, and abdomen. Its branches innervate a widespread range of body parts, from the head down to the abdominal organs, including the stomach. This nerve takes center stage in much of our autonomic nervous system, the portion of the nervous system that controls involuntary actions like your digestion, breathing, and heart's beating. You don't have to consciously think about these vital bodily activities; they happen on their own thanks to your autonomic nervous system and vagus nerve, which links the brain (and, in effect, your hypothalamus)

directly to your internal organs. In fact, in the yoga community, it is said that mastery over this nerve brings control over heart rate and digestion, as well as a high degree of control over pain. Breathing exercises typical of traditional yoga practice, for example, are believed to work directly with the vagus nerve, allowing an individual to change some of those involuntary, unconscious actions in the body. A classic example of this would be using a certain breathing exercise to modify the concentration of carbon dioxide in the blood, which can then influence the production of serotonin in the brain. Serotonin is among the brain chemicals that elicit feelings of euphoria and happiness. That said, for our purposes—simply put—when the top of your stomach is stretched out in response to a meal, the feeling of fullness is sent to your hypothalamus via the vagus nerve, a fast-track highway of information.

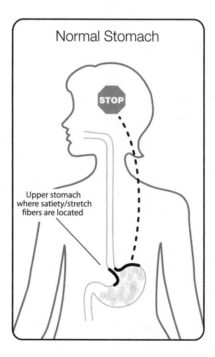

It should come as no surprise, then, that in all bariatric procedures the top 10 percent of the stomach area is maintained as the primary receptacle of food. It is here that the vagus nerve receives the stimulus that you are full. This is why my patients feel full on relatively small portions after surgery. They no longer have a lower 90 percent of a cavity to fill up first before the food reaches those sensors; the cardia is stretched out right away and fullness is sensed pretty immediately. You (who probably have not had such surgery) have the luxury of filling up the lower reaches of your stomach before feeling full. How do you gain control of the vagus nerve working with a fully intact stomach? I'll be getting to that in a moment, but let's finish the story here, because in addition to stretch receptors there are hormonal reactions that also occur. This is where ghrelin, leptin, and a protein called peptide YY come into play.

Other Messengers of Fullness: The two digestive hormones that share the remote control to your feelings of hunger and appetite are ghrelin and leptin. You may have heard about these hormones in recent years due to the volume of new research that has emerged about them. Studies in sleep medicine, for instance, have shown that when people are severely sleep deprived, they suffer an imbalance of these hormones, which then triggers an insatiable need to eat high-calorie foods. In essence, the brain fails to get the message that they are full, so they continue to eat.

As with many hormones in the body meant to achieve a balancing act and regulate certain biological processes, ghrelin and leptin are paired together but have opposing functions. One gives the green light to go and the other emits the red light that wants you to stop. Ghrelin (your "go" hormone) gets manufactured in the cells of the stomach and pancreas when your stomach is empty, and increases your appetite once the hypothalamus receives its transmission via the bloodstream that says, "I'm hungry. Feed me." Interestingly, ghrelin levels rise when people go on calorie-restriction diets, which may explain why dieting is so difficult. When people are injected with ghrelin and exposed to tantalizing food spreads, an area of the brain associated with addiction—one of its pleasure centers—lights up on brain scans more than it does in those who are not given the extra ghrelin. Because of ghrelin's interaction with not just the hypothalamus but also other areas of the brain related to pleasure, we know now that during times of stress ghrelin increases and may help with coping. Scientists at the University of Texas Southwestern Medical Center recently discovered that ghrelin has antidepressant and antianxiety effects in rodents. The consequence, though, for both rodents and humans is an increase in body weight from stress-induced eating.

Upon reaching fullness, fat cells secrete the other hormone—leptin (your "stop" hormone)—to transmit the "whoa" report to your hypothalamus so you can slow down and eventually avoid taking another bite. At this point ghrelin dramatically decreases so there are no mixed messages. When leptin was first identified, many scientists thought they had hit the jackpot: the skinny hormone. A flurry of experiments soon followed to capitalize on leptin's potential power over obesity. But upping leptin levels doesn't appear to help people shed weight. Obese people tend to already have increased levels of leptin circulating in their bloodstream, compared with leaner people, but can be resistant to its appetite-suppressing effects (not unlike the way type 2 diabetes is, in part, caused by a resistance to insulin). In other words, we cannot rely on leptin alone. Nor can we just focus on controlling ghrelin.

And then there is peptide YY, which is a short protein produced and released in the intestines. This protein increases the efficiency of digestion and nutrient absorption while the food moves through your GI tract. While we're not exactly sure how it works at the cellular level, peptide YY is thought to decrease appetite and, in turn, induce fullness. Attempts to use peptide YY directly as a weight-loss drug have been met with some success, but the jury is still out on whether a person can have a decreased sensitivity to this protein due to obesity. Research in just the last few years has shown that eating protein-rich foods can boost peptide YY levels naturally in the body, adding credence to why a high-protein meal like meat or poultry can bring on feelings of fullness much sooner than a high-carb one of pasta or rice. But it's important to realize that peptide YY—and leptin, and ghrelin—are just small links in the long chain of events that happens once your physical stomach receives food. For each of these hormones and feedback loops, there are at least 40 more that are thought to contribute, as either part of a pathway and/or as a potential standalone factor in our biology. Again, we have much to learn in this field. For now, a critical takeaway is that fullness originates in the stomach but culminates in the deepest, and perhaps most primitive, part of your brain. Zeroing in on these two "bookends" to the Full story can afford you a big advantage in taking control.

It takes about 20 to 30 minutes after you start eating for the crescendo of the effect of all these pathways, from your stretch receptors and vagus nerve to your appetite hormones and peptide YY, to hit the conscious part of you that acknowledges you're full. This is the point at which your hypothalamus is, by every definition of the word, full. If we are not mindful of this effect, we can eat through any reasonable sense of fullness and experience discomfort and malaise as a result (that is, that steakhouse or Thanksgiving aftermath).

The s-t-r-e-t-c-h of your stomach and your stomach's evaluation of what's in the food set off a nerve signal and hormone secretion sequence—the likes of which your body relishes. Your body treats the meal like the welcoming of the Publishers Clearing House "big-check" guy! Essentially all of your body systems are alerted to the meal and prepare to digest. This makes sense. Without the meal, nothing would be functioning. You wouldn't be here. In the wild, meals are king. And physiologically we have not changed much from this simple reality.

Sex, Drugs, Food . . . and Dope: The next phase in the body's experience of fullness is also rooted in an ancient internal wiring system. The euphoria that accompanies fullness is on par with a narcotic effect, and has been so for millennia. If you were to characterize this blissful feeling from a physical standpoint, you'd notice that while in this state, you look relaxed, your breathing has slowed, your pupils have dilated, and you report feeling happy. Along with sex, this is one of the few indulgences available to us naturally on a regular basis. The guilty party in this reaction is not, in fact, the food itself. But it's what the food does to the reward and pleasure system in the body—unleashing a rush of the feel-good neurotransmitter dopamine. Dopamine is your master of motivation, delivering intense feelings of enjoyment that can positively reinforce the behavior that stimulated the dopamine bath to begin with. In fact, many addictions to substances like cocaine, amphetamines, and alcohol are attributed to this response. These drugs target the same reward system—only much more powerfully. This helps explain why many narcotics abusers are pretty scrawny; their hypothalamic pleasure centers are gratified so they don't feel the need or desire for food. They have another, albeit dangerous, means by which to trigger their dopamine surges.

In addition, *what* you eat also can enhance this effect, as some nutrients in foods act as precursors to these neurotransmitters in the brain that can be very pleasurable. Carbohydrates, for example, are famous for triggering the release of serotonin that reduces pain and produces a sense of calm. Most prescription antidepressants are formulated to increase serotonin levels in the brain—to make you feel good. On the other hand, when proteins are broken down into their amino acid building blocks during digestion, one amino acid called tyrosine further increases the production of dopamine and dopamine's main precursors, norepinephrine and epinephrine, which increase levels of alertness and energy. (I'll be exploring what happens to food's components—proteins, fats, and carbohydrates—in digestion in the next chapter.)

To say this is a powerful system is an understatement. An unsatisfied brain is very unhappy, and you'll only be able to think about your hunger as would a famished, foraging reptile or hunting caveman. Have you ever tried to ignore your hunger? How productive were you then? It's not surprising that starving people throughout history have been known to eat their shoes, bugs, grass, each other. Regardless of intelligence or IQ, a person without appetite satisfaction (or, for a better way to put it, *fullness*) is a person without reason. Again, we have our preprogrammed hypothalamus to thank for that survival mechanism. You could be sitting in a five-star restaurant utilizing the most advanced, evolved areas of your brain in conversation and if your hypothalamus is not getting what it needs, it will not stop bothering you. Unfortunately, for those of us trying to control our weight, we rarely find ourselves facing starvation and instead, encounter the opposite: a bounty of highly accessible and palate-pleasing food that doesn't require us to exert much energy or effort to acquire (and consume). The pleasure-seeking hunger of early humans has translated into an obesity and diabetes epidemic in modern times. Our old brains just haven't evolved yet to deal with this problem of overload.

Though some people may like to think their brains are dysfunctional and can't ever get the message that they are full, this condition is extremely rare. Prader-Willi Syndrome (PWS) is a complex genetic disorder in which people experience a chronic feeling of hunger that often leads to excessive eating and life-threatening obesity. It affects approximately 1 in every 12,000 to 15,000 people. Due to an inherited abnormality on the 15th chromosome, leading to a dysfunctional hypothalamus, their primitive brains never get clued in to that feeling of fullness. Their urge to eat is physiological and overwhelming, and there is no cure. They cannot qualify for surgery because they wouldn't be able to respond to the "Full effect" that's required in all of my patients. People with PWS are best treated by a genetic medicine specialist who can help them be extremely vigilant about their eating patterns.

Chances are you've got a fully functioning messenger system no matter what you weigh. When you don't listen to your body's internal signals of fullness, and respond accordingly, you override the system. This is what happens during a dinner out with friends, or an afternoon on the couch watching football in front of pizza and beer. When you indulge and experience the many pleasant aspects of the occasion, you ignore your innate fullness sensors. Remember, unlike our inherent antistarvation mechanism, our antiobesity mechanism is more subtle. It's virtually impossible to neglect feelings of hunger, but it's easy to neglect feelings of fullness.

Given all this brain chemistry, it's easy to see why most celebrations revolve around food. At special meals and feasts, we all get high on food. Just thinking about your grand holiday dinner may get your brain revved up in anticipation. On a much smaller scale, though, in terms of everyday eating, food desire is like an alcoholic's need for drink. But the person who drinks too much can wean himself from alcohol and no longer use it. To live, we must continue to eat. Harder still, if you have food and weight issues, you have to retrain your body to eat reasonably. You have to reacquaint yourself with those subtle cues of fullness, which brings me to how my patients learn to do this following a bariatric procedure.

Anatomy of Fullness: Bariatric Basics in Brief

As I explained earlier, I have learned much from my bariatric surgery experience that's applicable to every person seeking weight control. I'll teach you how the surgery works—the mechanics and brain effect insofar as they pertain to you. This will reinforce the concepts we just explored, for the anatomy of fullness is the foundation upon which the success of bariatric medicine is based.

First, it helps to keep in mind that the patients in my practice who qualify for surgery are not like the majority of the population. They not only have a lot of weight to lose (usually at least 100 pounds or more), but they are genetically programmed to be obese; that is the chief reason why previous diets have never worked for them. They require a more dramatic intervention to manage their genetics so they can then reduce the set of serious health risks they bear with all that extra weight. By definition, the term *morbid obesity* is a medical condition in which excess body fat has accumulated to the extent that it has an adverse effect on health, leading to reduced life expectancy. They feel trapped in a body that cannot shed the weight no matter what they do. That is, until they consider an anatomical rearrangement.

There are two commonly accepted ways in which people lose weight through surgery: (1) the Roux-en-Y Gastric Bypass (also called "bypass" and "gastric stapling"—see Figure 1); and (2) restrictive, adjustable, gastric banding (in the United States, usually known as the Lap-Band or Realize Band—see Figure 2). For simplicity, I'll call the first "bypass" and the second "band." These are the procedures with the longest and most well-documented effectiveness and safety records, and will suffice for purposes of our discussion.

The bypass was originally applied as a weight-loss procedure in the 1960s, so it has a long track record, and new technologies over the years have vastly improved how this procedure is performed. Today, it's achieved laparoscopically, which is minimally invasive through very small incisions so there's a quicker recovery, less pain, and less risk of wound complications and infection. During the surgery, we reroute how food moves through the digestive tract by sidelining 90 percent of the stomach and keeping just the top 10 percent in the digestive stream. This small leftover receptacle area is called a pouch, and it's where all those stretch receptors lie to quickly trigger feelings of fullness. In addition to the bypass capitalizing on the stomach's cardia section, it also works because of the way we reconnect the pouch to the lower intestine bypass segment. By linking the pouch directly to the middle portion of the small intestine, bypassing the rest of the stomach and the upper portion of the small intestine, we can create a bottleneck effect as food slowly passes through bit

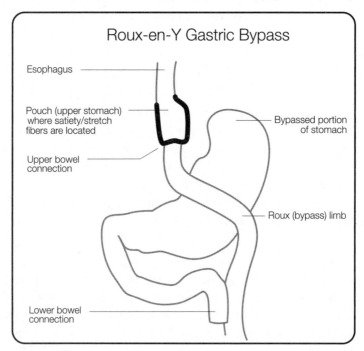

by bit. If food rushed through this connection, the stretch on the fullness fibers would be short-lived. Instead, the food is held in the pouch where it keeps it stretched, and a person stays full with a small meal for a longer period of time.

The factors that make the band work are similar to those of the bypass, with a few differences. The band is an inflatable silicone device that's wrapped around the upper part of the stomach to, again, preserve the uppermost cardia above the band. The band is connected by a tube to an access "port" that's fixed to the muscle wall just below the skin of the abdomen. By injecting water into this port via a thin needle through the skin, we can fill the band and make it narrower. By adjusting it in this manner, we can make the outlet from the upper stomach to the rest of the stomach smaller. As the band tightens, the emptying of food into the small intestine is slower and the upper stomach stays stretched with food for a longer period of time, which keeps a person feeling full longer.

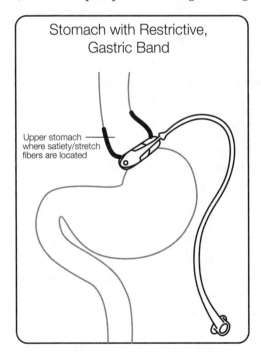

Stomach with Restrictive, Gastric Band

Upper stomach where satiety/stretch fibers are located

The risk of malnutrition is exceptionally rare in a band or bypass patient. In cases where it does happen, it almost always bespeaks a lack of follow-up and compliance. Bariatric patients typically reach a new, desirable, and steady state where their intake is more in line with their real metabolic needs, and they lose weight until this new balance is met. While they are encouraged to keep a specific nutritional supplementation regimen, it's very simple and limited. They eat less food, but the amount they eat post-surgery is ultimately all that they need to be healthy. And, most important, it's not their inner strength that gives them this control; it's their new wiring. It's their new tool. For the nonsurgical eater, again, it's not inner strength or willpower that keeps you at a healthy weight; it's using the tools.

The restriction with both procedures is essentially identical, as there are only two factors at play:

1. To feel full, you must stretch out the upper stomach and trigger the fullness fibers to signal your brain that you are full. (In the bypass, this is accomplished by filling the new pouch created, and in the band, this is done by filling the stomach above the band.)

2. To stay full, you must adjust how long the fullness fibers in your stomach stay stretched out. (In the bypass, this is achieved by keeping a small outlet from the pouch. In the band, this is done by adjusting the band itself to bring about slow emptying from the upper stomach.)

It's that simple. Clearly, in both procedures we are using a very small part of the potential size of the actual stomach. In the bypass, we have actually sectioned off most of the stomach and separated it away. In the band, we have segmented off the top part of the stomach above the band. The focal point in both procedures, however, becomes the cardia, where stretch receptors instigate whole-body fullness. The focal point for you, too, in taking control will be harnessing the power of your own cardia by using specific tools to prompt its fullness.

I cannot emphasize enough how definite and non-negotiable feelings of fullness are among my patients post-surgery. In support groups they joke about how many meals their anniversary dinner filet mignon lasted. And they are quick to remind me that prior to surgery, their appetites were often unstoppable. How much they ate before surgery was often very random and difficult to judge.

Postsurgical Tools

Why are my patients so successful after surgery? The critical difference is they now have a tool—that tool being their bypass or band, which helps them gain control of their portions and, in turn, their health. Their weight loss doesn't rely solely on this single tool, however. In addition to honoring their new anatomy, they must adopt other tools—other strategies—in their postsurgical life to continue and sustain the weight loss. And this is where the rubber meets the road for a lot of people. All of my patients receive what I call my "Rules of the Tool," which guides them through finding certain lifestyle strategies that help maximize the success of the bypass or band. Some of these tools will be the same ones I'll give you beginning in the next chapter. Prior to contemplating a single tool in your life, however, you must appreciate digestion and factor that into your overall strategy.

The Five Intentional Steps of Digestion

The first stages of digestion have very little to do with actually eating. They have real psychological and physiologic effects that have almost nothing to do with nutrition, but they get your mind and body ready to eat. The first part of your re-education is to recognize these elements as part of the eating process. They include (1) thinking about food, (2) smelling food, (3) tasting food, (4) chewing food, and (5) swallowing food. These are the "intentional" steps—the actions we can consciously control. Each discrete step is a point at which we can positively impact our dietary behaviors.

The first step—thinking about food—is relatively easy, and is usually accompanied by planning to eat. The best way to describe the power of the thinking-about-food stage is to consider what happens when you're a victim of a meal *denied*. This is a classic moment in my house as I have a ravenous, growing son. I'll have an amazing leftover meal waiting for me in the refrigerator, and I'll plan on eating it after a long day of surgery. While on my drive home, I'll have utilized my first stage of digestion—dreaming of what it will be like to sink my teeth into that particular meal. My mouth will even begin to water as it prepares for the experience. As is often the case, if my son has gobbled down all the leftovers, I'm then left with appetite dissatisfaction . . . stuck with the other (less desirable) food in my fridge. Not a happy moment.

In the next chapter, we'll come to see how certain tools can be applied here to this first step in the process, one of which entails having a premeal snack to take that ravenous hunger down a notch or two. Briefly, if you can preload the full experience *before* you eat a meal, then your hunger entering the meal can be notably decreased. You can come into a meal with your fullness processes already in motion, which is what I should have done on that drive home before finding out that my anticipated meal would not be what I expected.

The next three steps—smelling, tasting, and chewing—also relate to specific strategies you can use to maximize the Full effect. Without even going into the scientific details yet, you know from experience that foods that smell good and taste delicious are much more gratifying than their bland, boring counterparts. It's no wonder that eating a dozen rice cakes isn't enough to prevent someone from searching for better-tasting food nearby to literally fill a void. As you'll see, we must stimulate all of our gustatory centers.

The fourth step—chewing—is one of the most underestimated features of courting fullness, especially by those who try to lose weight by going on purely liquid diets. Chewing begins the digestive processes with action from the salivary glands in your mouth. This is where food breakdown commences both physically and biochemically. Liquid diets that abandon this step leave a gaping hole in the eating experience that can compel a person to eat more until that hole is filled. Anyone who has downed a shake or fruit smoothie and reached for a chewy snack soon afterward, regardless of how caloric that beverage was, knows what I mean. (I'll be giving you specific tools for incorporating shakes into your diet in the next chapter. You don't have to banish them from your life, but you do have to pay attention to the types of shakes you consume.)

In the fifth step—swallowing—your digestive tract is prepared for the abundance it's going to receive. There is a receptive relaxation of your lower esophageal sphincter and your stomach in anticipation of the food's delivery to your gut. There is also a physical fulfillment gained from the swallowing process—once again not experienced to any meaningful degree in those who drink all of their calories.

The result of all five intentional steps of digestion is food filling your stomach. As you know by now, this is where fullness becomes a concrete, nonnegotiable experience thanks to the constellation of events that take place among those stretch receptors, and the coinciding hormonal messengers that fire off to relay full signals to your primitive brain.

Your User's Manual

Recently, I was talking with a patient of mine who had bypass surgery two years ago. She had lost about 150 pounds in the first year and was about 10 pounds from her goal weight range. When she came to see me again at her two-year, post-surgery anniversary, she had gained back about 15 pounds of the 150 she had lost. Now she was 25 pounds away from her goal weight range.

She explained, "I just cannot stop eating a bag of chips and some chocolate every day. I have no control." No matter what I said, she still replied with, "I have no control." I looked at her and thought, *Hmm, no control?*

So I asked her a series of provocative questions to shake her up. "How often do you cheat on your husband? Do you drink to excess every day—getting falling-down drunk? Do you recklessly drive 100 miles per hour on the highway—cutting off cars and tailgating?" I thought she was going to kick me, and that her 25-year-old daughter who was with her was going to burst into hysterics. My patient was stunned and more than a bit offended.

"I've never done any of those things!" she said vehemently.

So I told her that I disagreed with her view of her limitations. I said, "It seems to me that you have a lot of control. You respect your marriage. You moderate your intake of alcohol. And you show good judgment on the road. On a daily basis you show a lot of control in the areas I mentioned." She smiled and got what I was hinting at. The problem was not her lack of control. The problem was that she did not think that having dietary control was important. After all she had put her family and friends through—the potential risk to her life and health if she didn't lose the weight, the monetary investment in surgery, and the stress of the operation and recuperation—why wasn't having dietary control still a priority?

I told her that she was being very unfair to herself and her family. Maybe even selfish. She thought hard about this, put it into perspective and left with a renewed faith in her ability to control her world. I also reminded her to listen to those cues of fullness. They are there, shouting every time, and all she had to do was tune into them. I also prescribed a few more tools to add to her regimen, including one that would allow her to enjoy potato chips and chocolate, her favorite "poisons," so messages of fullness would ring loud and clear.

There is a lot of uncertainty in life, so it's important to have some control where we can. And for those who are trying to manage their weight, it feels bad not to be in control. Why subject yourself to these feelings of failure?

Whether I'm talking to people who need to lose 200 pounds or those who would like to drop 20, the response I hear after I explain to them their innate need to appease the most primitive part of their brain is similar: they feel relieved to learn that a seeming lack of control is not due to their own personal shortcomings or weakness. There's no faulty wiring. There's no defect or muted brain. The truth is, you can't fool your primitive brain no matter how much you weigh or how smart you are. Let me give you another way to look at it.

Commonly Accepted Methods for Weight Loss among the Obese*

Strategy	Results
Diet	10% loss of excess body weight 67% of weight regained at 1 year
Exercise	5% loss of excess body weight
Behavior Modification	5% to 10% loss of excess body weight at 2 years
Antiobesity Drugs	5% to 10% loss of excess body weight (potential danger)

Summary of results: Approximately 10% weight loss in 1 to 2 years. After 5 years, most regain all weight that was lost. Morbidly obese regain 95% to 98% in fewer than 5 years.

The bottom line: Even in the most successful programs, 95% of these people regained all of their lost weight within 5 years.

*Source: National Institutes of Health Conference on Morbid Obesity, 1992

In all of my bariatric lectures, when I'm talking to candidates for surgery, I always present the 1992 NIH Consensus Conference Data about nonoperative treatments for morbid obesity, such as medications, exercise, dieting, behavioral therapy, and so on.

Everything *except* surgery. Before presenting the data, I say to the audience, "All of you are here because you don't know how to diet and exercise properly, right?" As expected, they all nod their heads in agreement. I then stop and make sure they understand that what I am about to show them is the most important slide they are ever going to see in their dieting career. The information they are about to learn is going to change the way they view their struggles and themselves—forever. I then say to the audience, "I can't believe you still believe that! After tens of years of dieting, and often tens of thousands of dollars spent, you still believe that you can't lose weight because you *don't know* how to eat properly and exercise? That's ridiculous!"

After I let the audience take in the sobering contents, I then go on to reiterate the limited effectiveness of well-known strategies like diet and exercise over a five-year period. Ninety-five percent of people cannot sustain weight loss for five years using any of these methods. Considering the fact that more than 95 percent of dieters in general cannot sustain weight loss in the long term, this discouraging news relates to both those who are morbidly obese and those who are just a little overweight. At this point in my presentation, everyone in the audience breathes a sigh of relief and some start to cry. They realize that their failure is expected, because the simple truth is that dieting doesn't work, even though many people are slow to believe it. Often I watch supporting spouses turn to their loved ones and apologize to them. They frequently say, "I'm sorry. I thought you just weren't following through. I thought you weren't committed. I didn't know."

There are few bets in life that you can win 95 percent of the time. For the non-morbidly obese dieter, someone with 10, 20, 40, 50 pounds to lose, the lessons also ring true. The diets you have tried are rarely effective in helping you lose and maintain weight loss. You are genetically programmed to fail on a diet, but you are not genetically programmed toward an inability to lose weight.

Fullness is in all of us. Grasping this internal wiring for fullness is like finishing a user's manual to a new gadget. Now you can use that knowledge (and wiring) to your advantage, which is the whole point of the tools, and of this book. Since the Stone Age, humans have employed tools to make life a little easier and to propel the human race forward with new technology. Why not employ special tools to make weight control effortless?

Let's get to them.

The Full Challenge: Day 3

One of the most powerful tools that you're going to learn more about in the upcoming chapters, and which plays upon the science of fullness described in this chapter, is how to take a more mindful approach to eating. You cannot appreciate or gain control of the five intentional steps of digestion—(1) thinking about food, (2) smelling food, (3) tasting food, (4) chewing food, and (5) swallowing food—unless you stop to really think about what you're doing every step of the way. Seizing control of these steps in a very conscientious manner will be the ultimate secret to your success. Once you learn how to perform these five functions, which are cognitive, sensorial, and physical, you'll automatically achieve that kind of effortless control over your weight that you've been dreaming about for a long time.

Let's start today with this process. See if you can identify all five intentional steps of digestion at every meal. At your first meal of the day, I want you to sit down and actually write out answers to each of these questions: How much do you think of the food before you eat? How does it smell? What does it taste like (try to use very descriptive terms—take time to really taste the food like you've never had it before)? What is the experience of chewing your food like? How does the food feel in your mouth? How do your feelings, from your emotional ones stemming from your brain to your deeply physiological ones streaming up from your gut, change as you swallow the food?

Perform this brief mental exercise every time you put something in your mouth today, including things you drink. Notice the experience of eating as a clearly defined moment from beginning to end. With every bite, you're changing how you think and how you feel. Tomorrow, make it a goal to be as mindful as you can every time you eat. The goal is for this to become a regular part of your eating experience. By paying extra attention to the steps of your eating routine, you can eventually create a new habit whereby you're always aware of your eating behavior and levels of fullness. This will ultimately help you to self-regulate how much you eat so that you keep your eating aligned with your true hunger.

ADAM BITTERMAN

Age: 45, Height: 5'7"
Starting: Weight: 218, Size: 38"
Final: Weight: 187.2, Size: 36"
Total Lost: 30.8 Pounds and 24"

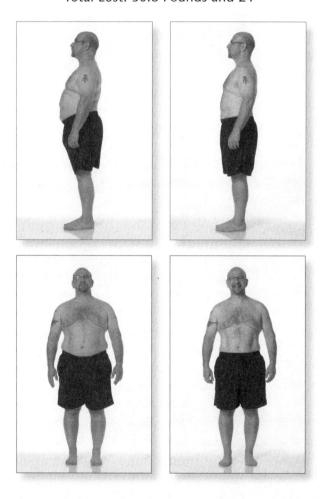

"When my doctor and girlfriend advised that I really needed to lose weight, I took it seriously. But I was nervous because I'd tried everything from Nutri-System to food delivery. The weight crept up when I got a desk job seven years ago, and I noticed that my metabolism has dropped since turning 40. I'm from Chicago, and I love food! I'm well on my way to reaching my target weight loss of 40 pounds. I feel great, and people are starting to notice my weight loss."

BUILDING YOUR FULL TOOLBOX

Tools are critical to our success in so many areas in our life—e-mail and cell phones to communicate, Internet to research, cars to get to where we are going, and so on. Why would we think that we don't need such help with our weight-loss efforts? As the previous chapter pointed out, the big secret that I have learned from my experiences in weight-loss surgery is that success lies in having a tool. My patients leave the operating room with the tool of a bypass or band. But, like any tool, it is no more effective than the person using it. Even a bypass or band cannot guarantee success, though it does give a person a tremendous advantage over their old self. Similarly, the tools I'll be giving you can equip you with the edge over that primitive, reptilian brain that constantly seeks fullness, and that is constantly confronted with an abundance of food.

Just recently, I had a patient come to see me who had gained back about 40 pounds of the 160 pounds she had lost five years ago. She had not been compliant with follow-up and was mad at me because I "allowed her to gain weight back." In reviewing her history of the past four-plus years, we stumbled on the fact that her diet, meal volume, and activity levels were not commensurate with a maintained weight loss. She was eating poorly and not being active in any way. When I pointed out this (obvious) set of issues, her retort was, "Why did I bother having surgery if I had to do all of that?" I was aghast that she had forgotten the mantra of those who have bariatric surgery—that I will give you the starting tool that then allows you to work the other tools! Bariatric patients don't suddenly become immune to weight-control efforts. My patients still have to work at it like everyone else. The surgery simply places my patients on a level field.

Imagine her disappointment when her denial mechanisms allowed her to forget her first year's post-op successes. It was her own work! And, not surprisingly, when we got her back on track she flourished once again, just by following my guidelines (what I call "the Rules of the Tool") for making her new anatomy work for her.

When I talk about tools to lose or control your weight, keep in mind: there is no one tool set for everyone. I like to give you a mix of different tools so you can see which fits best with you and your life. The tools outlined in this chapter reflect the "best of the best"—the ones that the vast majority of my patients have found to be very helpful in their weight-loss journey. None of these tools are truly revolutionary, but each one is simple, practical, customizable, and will make you feel like you're in control of your dietary life without being on a proverbial diet. Do not try them all at once. Do not implement even half in your life right away. Just add one or two in slowly and make a commitment to the process.

A key question to ask yourself is this: what can you modify, add on, and work with that doesn't feel drastic or leave you deprived? There is really no shortcut to the economics of weight loss and management. It is all about calories in and calories out. The secret is to work with what you can do relatively easily. Most people gain weight because of the aggregate effect of lots of small changes over time, such as graduating from school and stopping sports (but continuing to eat as always), having a stressful job and no time to make meals, and having a child and no time for routine workouts. Many of my patients did not gain their excess 100 pounds overnight. These pounds were often gained over decades of slow, steady weight gain. They often can pinpoint the time in their lives when their weight started to be an issue, such as after an injury or once they turned 30 and got married. Although quite a number of my patients have "always been big," many note a pivotal moment in their lives when the balance of weight control over obesity was lost. It's not that they suddenly stopped caring about their weight. Rather, an insidious process started that they were powerless to reverse. The good news is that we approach losing the weight by making lots of small changes over time. Just as glacial changes are responsible for much of the world's topography (think of Yosemite National Park), minuscule changes in your life can effect a massive outcome.

First, I'll present a few ground rules for choosing and applying the tools, emphasizing again that it's virtually impossible to use all the tools at once (I know that some of you will try anyway). Remember, the goal here is to simply pick one or two tools to start and then experiment with others to figure out which ones fit best. Any combination of these tools can be extremely effective.

What Kind of Results Can You Expect?

My goal for you is to lose one to two pounds a week. Studies have found that rate to be sensible, safe, and sustainable. It's also just enough to keep you engaged and believing in your body's system. Surely, if you adopt the principles here, a greater weight loss is possible, but once again, I don't want to set you up for failure. You may be disappointed that I'm not promising you thin thighs in 30 days, washboard abs in a week, or size 4 skinny jeans in a month. But remember all the times you were promised such miracles, and how each ended in failure? A simple one-pound weight loss a week over a year equals a 52-pound total loss. Half a pound every week for a year is 26 pounds lost. Obvious and simple math, but when it hits home, you see the profound effect of what I'm talking about. Now, to maintain that loss is notable for most of us. That modest weight loss is the minimum of what I'm shooting for. And consider how such a loss could affect your life: I want you to feel like you're eating "normally." I want you engaged in your life, including being able to eat like a "real person." I want you to be in control and I want you to taste the success that comes from living within reason and moderation. There's no substitute for enjoying high self-esteem and avoiding the constant cycle of failure.

I realize that there's a group of you who is approaching this with the following mentality: *Here comes another chance to prove that I'm destined to be fat; I'm big-boned and I look like everyone in my gene pool.* There is clearly a genetic and physiologic component to where your body is set right now. More than anyone, as a bariatric surgeon who treats people with morbid obesity every day, I understand how genetics and biological makeup come into play. But I also know small steps over time make a big difference and can give you ultimate control regardless of your personal built-in challenges. I've witnessed it firsthand thousands of times.

Look at your own experience. You've done diet programs that have given you short-term control and failed because they asked too much of you. When you revert to your old eating habits, the weight comes back. Between the two is a happy middle ground that I'm confident you can find. What do you have to lose by considering this option?

We all think that if it's not painful, it's not going to work and it's not worth doing. That's a very American sentiment. We are so engaged in the drama and the sacrifice and the all-or-nothing mentality. Let's not do that when it comes to maintaining our weight and health from now on. Take it one tool at a time, starting with two simple ground rules.

Ground Rule #1: Do Not Start on Monday

When you begin a life change, the temptation is to have a target start date. Classically, this is "next Monday." It hints at a change so disruptive and difficult that you have to prepare for it. I am not a fan of such disruption and planned orchestration. Any change that you will stick with requires only that you begin. As the often overquoted saying goes, "A trip of a thousand miles begins with one step." Well, that step is not so hard to take and the process of beginning any monumental journey of transformation should be similarly easy. So, find what hints and tools you can add now without any preparation or organization. Do not wait. Add them now. As in, before you go to bed tonight.

Ground Rule #2: Do Not Make It Hard Like You Always Have

I've said this already, but it bears repeating. When we try to transform ourselves, we usually feel the need to change everything, and all at once. It's hard for my patients to understand that that is never my intention. Just recently I had a patient I'll call Jane who lost 120 pounds following her Lap-Band placement a year ago. She has about 30 pounds to go to reach her goal range. I reviewed her diet history and found that she was not doing any physical activity whatsoever and she had made potato chips a big part of her everyday life again. When I asked Jane about her questionable exercise and food choices, she told me that she was going to get a trainer three days per week, cut out all processed carbs, and do an additional hour of aerobics every day. I stopped her mid-sentence, partially appalled and partially exhausted from listening to her overwhelming plan. I said, "It's not going to work." Jane was disheartened and felt that I had lost faith in her. I told her nothing was further from the truth. In fact, I felt that she had done wonderfully, but that she would not be able to execute this plan and, most probably, the disappointment at the failure would ultimately make her change nothing.

Jane realized that I was right. She was taking my simple suggestions and making them too hard. (It's how we do dieting in America!) Why does it always have to be a clean sweep or a total life makeover? That's not realistic. I told Jane to walk one mile four days per week and add a quarter mile every week. By her next appointment in eight weeks she would be doing almost three miles four days per week. In addition, I told her to eat only one measured cup of potato chips once on the weekend and twice per week—a total of three times per week (as opposed to her eating multiple bags per week). I showed her how this would probably result in about a three- to four-pound loss per month. (I'll explain how to apply this "cheat prescription" to your personal plan in Chapter 6.) In three short months, she would be down 9 to 12 pounds with just this simple step. And by next summer, she would be within her goal range. She said, "That sounds so easy." I reassured her that it was, as it should be.

So don't make this process difficult by weighing yourself down—literally—with unrealistic expectations. You may find it relatively easy to initially instigate several shifts in your routine and dietary habits, but then struggle farther down the road. I'd rather see you start slowly and build momentum over time. Remember, take this one tool at a time.

The Tools

Tool #1: Be Full with Less

Bread. Pasta. Rice. Potatoes. Chips. Crackers. Doughnuts. Bagels. Baked goods. I know you can eat a lot of this "white stuff" because it's physiologically easy to do. Gram for gram, they contain more calories than other types of foods and their ingredients don't work well with your body's biology to signal when you've had enough (that is, they don't tell your brain that you're full soon enough).

One of the secrets to keeping your ability to sense fullness is to eat bulky foods, especially those with some protein and fiber. It's far easier to eat your way through a fresh bread basket than to chow down an equivalent amount of calories in sweet peppers. But you'll feel a sense of fullness much quicker as you chew on the sweet peppers. Not only do bell peppers contain a lot of water and fiber (hence, they are typically "high-volume" foods, supplying the most food with the fewest calories), but the act of chewing the peppers takes time and effort that also factors into your fullness equation. Recall in the previous chapter how the act of chewing plays a key role in reaching fullness. The longer a food needs to be chewed, the shorter it usually takes for it to contribute to your sense of fullness.

Now, I'm not asking you to suddenly ditch all bread in favor of sweet peppers. I know that's not realistic. But choosing high-volume as opposed to concentrated, calorie-dense foods can help you trim your caloric intake without trimming your sense of fullness. You may even feel *fuller* when you're actually eating *less*.

Remember, anything with the words "enriched flour" in the ingredients calls for a pause. These foods are not evil, but they do pack a powerful punch of calories in a small and usually unfulfilling portion. Most of these represent processed foods that were developed in food manufacturing plants to give "cheap and easy" calories with minimal effort. While they serve a function for physically demanding times, like when preparing for a marathon, for most of us, they slowly poison our metabolism. We have no need for this amount of calories that are so easy to consume. I don't expect you to banish these from your life entirely, but I do encourage you to minimize them while maximizing foods manufactured wholly by nature. I like foods that look the same as they did before man got a hold of them.

Full on Fiber: You've probably noticed that fiber has gotten its own public relations team lately. Food manufacturers will tout the benefits of their product's fiber content if they can (and sometimes when they shouldn't if the grams of fiber are ridiculously low). This is all for good reason, as a growing body of scientific research continues to prove the benefits of fiber for heart health, disease prevention, and weight control. Emerging research shows how fiber can lower bad (LDL) cholesterol, blood pressure, the risk for developing diabetes and some types of cancer, and help people to lose weight. Women need to get at least 25 grams of fiber a day;

men should aim for 30 grams a day. A lot of us fall far short of these targets. Some studies suggest that consuming an *extra* 14 grams of fiber per day (a total of 39 to 44 grams per day) may cause the body to absorb 10 percent fewer calories.

Fiber comes in two forms, soluble and insoluble, and it's good to get a balance of both. Soluble fiber dissolves in water and is found mostly in nuts, seeds, legumes (beans, lentils, peas), fruit, and oat bran. It's the "digestible" fiber that helps lower your risk for heart disease and can lower bad cholesterol. Insoluble fiber, on the other hand, does not dissolve in water so it's this "indigestible" form. Found mostly in whole grains and vegetables, it passes through your body and literally acts like a broom through your system, pushing food along and aiding in digestive health.

It helps to think of fiber as a traffic cop. It allows your digestion to reach an ideal speed that supports optimal metabolism and, ultimately, fullness. Just as all foods are not created equal, not all foods get digested at the same speed. Nutrients from certain foods get in your bloodstream at different times, which changes the chemistry of hormones that either make you feel full or stimulate you to want more food. Insulin in particular, the pancreatic hormone that spikes when you're eating carbohydrates, guides glucose from the blood to the cells. It's largely responsible for making you feel hungry for more when you've eaten quickly digested foods, such as white bread and fruit juice. Simple carbohydrates take only five to ten minutes to get absorbed. Foods that make you feel full, though, take longer to get into the system, somewhere between 30 minutes to two hours, depending on the food's makeup. This ideal window of 30 minutes to two hours happens when you eat proteins, and high-fiber veggies, fruits, and whole grains, which help prevent insulin surges and maintain a healthy blood-sugar balance.

So fiber becomes a key player in creating a meal that will get digested slowly, and as such, is less likely to be quickly converted to fat and stored. For instance, in the presence of fiber, plain old sugar will get released more gradually into the bloodstream than if it were by itself. In fact, you can combine a quickly digested food such as white bread with a slow one that has fiber and change how your body responds. For example, if you spread a nut butter on top of a bagel, the fiber and fat in the nut butter will prevent the glucose from getting rapidly digested. Similarly, a mix of fibrous veggies in a bowl of pasta will change the "chemistry" of the whole dish.

Fiber-rich foods also tend to be bulky, which, as I said, promotes fullness. You can reduce your calories but not how full you feel just by adding more fibrous vegetables to a meal. For example if you make lasagna with lots of asparagus and mushrooms, bite for bite you'll consume fewer calories and get to that sense of fullness much sooner than if you were to eat a classic cut of meat and cheese lasagna.

Following is a list of high-fiber foods broken down into three tiers. I've created these separate categories because there's a difference between eating a cup of kale versus a cup of rice, even if it's brown rice. Choose from Tier I as often as you like; these are your all-star vegetables that will make you full on less due to their fiber and water content. Tier II includes fruits, which also have fiber and volume but a higher concentration of sugar (and thus calories). When you eat from Tier II, be sure you're eating the whole fruit and not just the juice! Any fruits with edible skins, such as apples and berries, are great choices because the skins contain fiber too. Tier III includes the grains and starchy vegetables, which are dense in calories but have a Full effect due to their high fiber content.

Reminder: Avoid strict diets and misery. Concentrate on simple tools you can do and live with over time. Choose only the tools that will fit into your life.

Tier I (high-volume vegetables and fruits)		
artichoke	cucumber	romaine lettuce
arugula	green beans	spinach
asparagus	kale	sugar snap peas
broccoli	mushrooms	summer squash
Brussels sprouts	mustard greens	tomato
cauliflower	onion	turnips
celery	peas	water chestnuts
chard	red and green cabbage	zucchini
collard greens		
Tier II (medium- to low-volume vegetables and fruits)		
apple	cherries	peach
apricot	dates	pear
banana	grapefruit	pineapple
beets	kiwi	plum
berries (especially blackberries, raspberries, blueberries)	mango	prunes
	nectarine	pumpkin
	orange	rutabaga
cantaloupe	papaya	sweet pepper
carrots	parsnips	watermelon
		winter squash
Tier III (grains and starchy vegetables)		
beans (black, pinto, kidney, garbanzo, lima)	eggplant	whole-grain bread
	lentils	whole-grain cereals
bran cereals	oatmeal	whole-grain crackers
brown rice	potato	whole-grain tortillas
butternut squash	quinoa	whole-wheat couscous
corn	split peas	whole-wheat pasta
	sweet potato or yams	

Full Power of Protein: Anyone who has ever eaten a large cut of beef or chicken knows the full power of protein. It's much easier to put your fork down when you've had your fill of protein, even in the presence of carbohydrates, than if you're only eating a bowl of pasta. This is partly due to the fat content that often accompanies protein (and I'll explain why fat is so satisfying shortly), but it's also a result of how much effort it takes your body to break down and utilize protein. Proteins are comprised of amino acids, the "building blocks of life." When consumed, your body goes to work breaking down proteins into their amino acids, which then get absorbed and transported by the blood to cells for use. The mere act of breaking down protein burns calories and keeps your blood sugar stabilized. Amino acids can then be converted to glucose and used as energy or they can form new protein molecules needed by the body, including those that build, repair, and support muscle tissue. They are also involved in a variety of bodily functions, such as growing hair and nails, creating enzymes and hormones, and maintaining the health of your internal organs and blood.

Amino acids are required to break down fat, too. Specifically, protein consists of 22 amino acids, 11 of which are essential so you have to get them from foods because your body can't manufacture them on its own. A couple of these essential amino acids play a critical role in feeding the energy units of cells, called the mitochondria. Just as water facilitates the transportation of molecules in the body, so does protein. For fat cells to open their doors and let the fat out to be burned as fuel, protein and water must be present.

After my patients have bariatric surgery, I want them to get full with the most reasonably sized meals possible. Their nutritional needs must also be met with these much smaller meals, too. In this regard, protein is king. Its density allows my patients to be full relatively quickly in their surgically created small stomachs. And protein's density also slows down the emptying of the pouch, thus keeping them full longer. The power of protein in your life will be similar. You can achieve fullness with less food, and the fullness will be more intense so you'll stay full longer.

Think of this from your own past experience. Again, compare the fullness effect differences between a steak or chicken breast and a plate of pasta. I can almost guarantee it takes a lot less volume of protein to make you full than with a meal comprised of mostly carbohydrates. You couldn't eat a whole mound of steak, but you could probably put down a box of pasta. Recall, too, the difference in your fullness between these two meals. The old joke of how people are hungry an hour after eating Chinese food is not far from the truth. The noodle and rice dishes cannot hold your hunger and maintain your fullness the same way compact protein can. Sure, there are other metabolic factors at play, but from a purely bulk-and-density perspective, protein's power to trigger fullness is non-negotiable.

Having a steady intake of protein throughout the day will help you avoid cravings and increase your feelings of fullness, so you feel less hungry between meals. I don't expect you to turn into a carnivorous protein hound, but if you can aim to make lean proteins one-third of your meals, you'll stretch out that upper part of the stomach and trigger that full feeling quickly. And therein lies the challenge: focusing on *lean* proteins and lightening up on heavy, fatty proteins that are calorie dense. Below is a guide to help you choose your proteins carefully. Although dairy typically contains a combination of carbohydrates, fat, and protein, I've included it here since most dairy products contain a healthy amount of protein.

Lean Proteins
Eggs
Low-fat cheeses
Most fish* (clams, cod, flounder, halibut, mahimahi, mussels, orange roughy, salmon, scallops, sea bass, shellfish, shrimp, snapper, sole, swordfish, trout, tuna [fresh or canned in water], yellowtail)
Nonfat and low-fat cottage cheese
Nonfat and low-fat milk
Nonfat and low-fat yogurt
White meat chicken and turkey (no skin)

*Though different fish contain different amounts of fat—salmon, for instance, is a high-fat fish compared with flounder—the fat in most coldwater fish is loaded with omega-3 fatty acids (the "good fat" your brain and body crave) so you needn't worry so much about consuming too much. Besides, it's hard to eat too much fish!

Medium- to High-Fat Proteins		
Bacon	Hot dogs	Roast beef
Dark meat chicken and turkey	Lamb	Salami
	Liver	Steak
Duck	Pork	Turkey sausage
Ground beef	Regular dairy (regular milk, cheeses, and yogurt)	
Ham		

Not all calories are created equal. In theory, a calorie is a calorie. But from a practical standpoint based on how the body responds to calories from different sources, not all calories are necessarily "equal." A candy bar, for example, is chock-full of refined sugar and unhealthy fat that will likely get stored in your fat cells. There's new evidence to show that ingredients in some foods can also disrupt your metabolism and your hormonal system, which impacts how well your body processes and burns energy. A class of natural and synthetic chemicals known as endocrine-disrupting chemicals (EDCs), also gaining the name "obesogens," can act in a variety of ways to make and keep you fat: by mimicking human hormones such as estrogen, by misprogramming stem cells to become fat cells, and, researchers think, by altering the function of genes. They enter our bodies also through a variety of ways: from natural hormones found in soy products, from hormones administered to animals, from plastics in some food and drink packaging, from ingredients added to processed foods, and from pesticides sprayed on produce. The lesson: when you eat minimally processed natural foods, you help stoke your body's metabolism so you can burn more fat.

Tool #2: Stop and Think

"Mindful" eating is easier said than done. But one of the keys to being more aware of your eating habits and that elusive feeling of fullness is to honor those five steps of digestion I discussed in Chapter 3. Every meal or snack should meet all five criteria. In other words, a food must allow you to experience thinking, smelling, tasting, chewing, and swallowing. All of these steps happen before one calorie is absorbed by the body, but they are critical components of the process. Remember that for this reason, I do not advocate liquid-only diets. If you are going to use shakes as part of your dietary regimen, make sure that they follow my framework of having at least 50 percent of their calories from protein (about 12.5 grams of protein per 100 calories), at least 5 grams of fiber, and a reasonable amount of calories (between 200 and 400). Also, be careful about using any of the body-building shakes. Not only can they contain too many calories, but some have been shown include a frightening level of contaminants like lead because they are based on chemical-laden formulations. (For more exceptions to this rule, as well as a great shake recipe see sidebar on the next page. Additional details on mindful eating will be described in Chapter 5.)

Cravings for salty and/or sugary foods—which are usually high in fat, too—can be extremely powerful, especially once your taste buds get a sampling. The last time you had salted potato chips or sweet and salty kettle corn, chances are you had more than one helping. Your taste buds will compel you to keep eating what recently stimulated them, so the more calorie-dense foods you eat, the more you'll want to eat them. These foods make it harder to go back to nutrient-rich foods no matter what your mind thinks and knows it should or shouldn't eat in copious amounts. This is why focusing on nutritionally dense foods from the start rather than trying to break the cycle of craving nutrient-poor foods is important to maximize weight loss, as well as for sustained energy and keeping your fullness center on cue.

To Shake or Not to Shake: There have been plenty of diets based on shakes, even for those who aren't trying to lose weight. Shakes have become a part of our dietary lexicon. They can be added to a sensible meal plan as long as they do not routinely take the place of eating regular, balanced meals. Just as all foods are not to be part of your everyday life, all shakes are not necessarily good for you. Some are no more than melted popsicles, ice cream, or candy bars. Read labels and make sure that they respect the balance of carbohydrates, proteins, fiber, and fats that I recommend. Look for all-natural ingredients. Rather than shakes based on ice cream and fruit juice, look instead for shakes that contain real yogurt, soy or whey protein powder, whole fruit, skim or low-fat milk (soy and almond milk are good, too), and healthy fats from wheat germ, flaxseed oil, or ground flaxseed. That said, be aware that even a "healthy" shake can be very rich in calories, so you wouldn't necessarily want this to accompany a regular meal as your beverage of choice. One of the best options for knowing that you're eating a healthy shake is to make your own. Below is one of my favorite recipes:

In a blender combine:

½ cup plain, fat-free yogurt

½ cup skim milk

1 scoop of low-calorie protein powder (look for a protein powder that contains at least 15 grams of protein per scoop; this can be any flavor—vanilla, chocolate, or strawberry)

2 teaspoons flaxseed

½ banana

1 cup fresh or frozen berries

1 cup ice

Place all ingredients in a blender and blend until smooth. Want a thicker shake? Add more ice!

For variations on the same theme, try different combinations of raspberries, blueberries, strawberries, pineapple, mango, coconut, etc. Frozen fruit options are a fantastic alternative to always having fruit around for shakes.

And I apologize for telling you something you probably already know (and might have tried before), but I implore you to make this a household rule: stay away from the television when you eat. When it comes to crippling your innate sense of fullness, I can't think of anything worse than eating in front of the television. When you're tuned into the television (or computer for that matter), you put yourself at a huge disadvantage because you're tuning out the channel between your stomach and brain. Scientific research bears this out.

A recent study at Yale University found that TV watchers who viewed snack commercials were inspired to eat just about anything (not just the brand featured). This snacking was totally unrelated to feeling either hungry beforehand or full afterward! In a 2006 study published in *Physiology and Behavior*, when people were exposed to television for 30 minutes, they consumed 36 percent more calories of pizza, or 71 percent more calories of macaroni and cheese, compared with people who listened to music for a half hour. In full fairness, listening to music also has been associated with higher food intake, but less so than watching television. And we can assume that people would eat the least if they weren't exposed to either television or music.

In general, people who keep their weight in check have been documented to watch far less television than those who struggle with their weight. The majority of people in the National Weight Control Registry, for instance (again, this is a group of about 5,000 people who have kept off at least 30 pounds over the long run), average about ten hours of television per week. Meanwhile, most people average about four hours per *day*.

So it's a foregone conclusion: separate eating from viewing electronic media, which includes your television and computer. I bet that if you just try to cut back on your digital engagements, and you don't do anything else differently (including altering what you eat), you'll still come out ahead because you'll become more physically active. Yet another recent study published in the *Archives of Internal Medicine* found that people who watched half as much TV as usual for three weeks burned an extra 119 calories per day. That's comparable to the effect of walking more than a mile.

If you must snack in front of the TV, choose your snacks wisely. Natural popcorn and raw veggies with a yogurt-based dip can fill you up without loading you down.

Create Discipline in the Home: Boundaries Set by a Mere Table: In an insightful essay for *The Wall Street Journal,* British physician Dr. Anthony Daniels wrote about the inherent boundaries established by having formal family meals, which are sadly rare these days. He wrote: "Family and social meals are among the most powerful teachers of self-control. They teach that the appetite of the moment is not, or rather ought not to be, the sole determinant of one's behavior. The pattern of grazing or foraging independently of everyone else teaches precisely the opposite lesson. It is hardly surprising that those who do not experience family or social meals early in life exhibit the lack of self-control that underlies so much modern social pathology in the midst of plenty."

To clarify, the "grazing and foraging" that Dr. Daniels talks about relates to the fact that people—especially children—have grown accustomed to nibbling mindlessly all day long on a surfeit of instantly gratifying foods high in fat and sugar. Unlike our hunter-gatherer ancestors who faced a scarcity of food, we have constant access to food and therefore we frequently never learn the discipline of controlling our appetites.

To this end, I challenge you to make family meals a priority. Designate certain days of the week when your family gathers around the table to eat together. Not only will your waistline enjoy the benefits, but so will your children's. Teach them how to cook and embrace the act of eating around the table as a social activity. The sooner they establish mindful eating practices, the better off they will be in leading a healthy, lean life.

Tool #3: Don't Fear Fat, but Don't Add Fat Either

I am not a "no-fat" guy. Your body needs fats to survive and make the essential hormones that keep our cells talking to one another. Also, your brain is largely fat and it needs to be kept alert if you are going to keep tricking it into being full (as I am recommending throughout this book). Body fat is not made by eating fat. It is the result of the wrong types of food and taking in too many calories in any form. Fat intake is not the enemy. Some fats are so important to your existence that they are called "essential fats." Essential fatty acids (EFA), specifically the omega-3 and omega-6 family of EFAs, are involved in biological processes and are necessary for survival. These healthy fats help fat-soluble vitamins like A, D, E, and K get around the body, create sex hormones, lower bad (LDL) cholesterol while elevating good (HDL) cholesterol, affect mood and inflammation, and contribute to the health of skin, eyes, nails, and hair. They also increase the satiety value of a meal, keeping you satisfied and feeling full.

So, how do you manage this dilemma of wanting to lose fat but not knowing how to eat fat? Well, my rule is to eat normal amounts of fat in your everyday life. Don't add fats to your diet. But don't avoid them, either. As an example, it is fine to cook with olive oil. But avoid eating a bag of full-fat chips or fried foods with any regularity. A handful of walnuts, which are rich in omega-3 fatty acids, is better than a handful of fatty crackers with a block of full-fat cheese. If it "seems" like a food is a fat indulgence, then it probably is. Do you need me to tell you to minimize funnel cakes? French fries? Doughnuts? I didn't think so.

Fats are also rich in flavor. A portion of our taste enjoys and needs fat to be satisfied. On some level, they give the brain satisfaction that it craves. To eliminate fats is to have a tasteless, dissatisfying diet. So maintain fats for flavor in moderation. And you'll still be able to court that taste satisfaction that you crave. I'd rather you eat the "right" food with a little bit of fat for flavor than eat the right foods in which you've eliminated all fat and flavor. Remember, too, that you can add a lot of flavor to foods just by reaching for extra spices, herbs, and citrus. Use more lemon, balsamic vinegar, cilantro, curry, garlic, ginger, ground pepper, light soy sauce, and mustard, for example, in your meals to liven them up!

When I tell you that fats are acceptable, as a physician I do need to at least make you aware of the difference between the types of fats. The healthier fats are the unsaturated fats. These are less likely to spend a lifetime lining your arteries. Foods that contain these fats include avocado, nuts, cold-water fish, flaxseed, chia seeds, pumpkin seeds, sunflower seeds, and vegetable oils such as canola and olive. The fats to limit are the saturated and trans fats. You can recognize these because they are in a solid state at room temp (think margarine, butter, lard, mayonnaise). These are used in many of the processed foods that we eat. They also have some effect in maintaining their taste and palatability over time. I really don't want to encourage you to be an obsessive label reader, but if you feel that something is too delicious to be good for you, check out the amount of saturated and trans fats.

> Remember, the fat in your diet is not the same as the fat on your body. Dietary fat and body fat are two very different things; excess body fat is the combined result of inactivity and over-eating any nutrients—proteins, carbohydrates, and fats. While most people could benefit from cutting back on their dietary fat intake, it's unhealthy to completely eliminate it from the diet.

Tool #4: Lighten Up on Liquid Pounds, and Think Water

Americans get 7 percent of their calories from soda. Stated another way, the average American consumes 50 gallons each year of sugar-sweetened beverages. No wonder cutting just one regular soda a day will melt away 20 pounds in a year (even if a person does nothing else). Maybe you feel you can't stop drinking your daily sodas, juices, double lattes, and sports drinks, but you can at least minimize them by dropping at least one a day or every other day. Keep the maximum number of calories from a drink to 70 to 100 calories, and watch your serving size. That bottle you're drinking may have 2.5 servings in it. Once you get into the habit of drinking more water, you'll feel lost without it. It takes a conscious effort to ensure you consume an adequate volume, but the health benefits are epic. And this is the easiest and least expensive thing you can do to support your health.

There are lots of low-calorie drinks on the market today, and you can create your own blends by simply mixing sparkling water and the juice from a lemon, lime, or orange. If you must have some juice, dilute an unsweetened juice drink such as cranberry, apple, or orange juice with sparkling water. Brew your own tea (any kind you want) and chill it down with ice. And remember, there's nothing wrong and a lot right with plain old water.

Water intake is a critical component of any weight-loss strategy. Aim to drink about 1.5 liters (approximately 52 ounces) per day. About 8 ounces every time you eat is perfect (with additional intake as needed to accompany any activity). This is the bare minimum I recommend. Water will help all of your body functions work more efficiently and it helps to flush out the waste products that are created by your body. The rule should be that your urine may have color in the morning. But as the day progresses, it should significantly clear up. The intake of water naturally starts to trigger your stomach's stretch satiety mechanism. This takes effort! Try it. Next time you are hungry, drink a glass of water and wait 20 minutes. Then see if you're somewhat less hungry. There is science behind how this works.

Why Water Is So Critical: Our bodies are about 75 percent water. Water helps keep your overall metabolism, fat metabolism, and all other bodily processes functioning properly. What's more, if the water content in your blood drops below normal, your muscle cells will leach water to support the flow necessary in the blood. When this happens, you become dehydrated. The first sign of this is hunger, and when they really need water, most people go for food, which can further lead them toward dehydration. Diets that severely restrict carbohydrates may give people the illusion of sudden weight loss, but here's why: cutting off carbohydrates forces the body to find other sources of energy. It likely turns to glycogen, which is stored carbohydrates on reserve in your muscles and liver. Once glycogen storages are tapped, water gets released. So someone who cuts back on carbs and notices sudden weight loss could be shedding just water weight rather than real fat weight. This could then prompt further dehydration and undeniable hunger.

Water is also a critical component of normal bowel habits. People who are challenged to drink enough water are often dehydrated and constipated. It takes two major dietary elements to stay regular: plenty of fiber *and* adequate hydration. One of the powers of insoluble fiber is to hold water in your lower bowels. Both fiber and water are critical for bowel movements. Not to get too graphic here, but when I used to do a lot of hemorrhoid surgery, I always prescribed more water and fiber to help with regularity. It's simple and cheap medicine.

What I love about telling patients to drink more water is that the advice has value without it costing anything or requiring a huge effort to follow. Water is such a perfect treatment for what may ail you, and, by definition, drinking water doesn't require much label reading, if any. It's calorie- and additive-free.

There's another aspect to this water equation. Not only do fat cells need water to convert fat to usable forms of energy, but your muscles also need water to perform. So when you increase your physical activity, your muscles will store more glycogen with water to meet the demands you're placing on them. Likewise, your bloodstream will carry more water, upping the amount of blood traveling through your system to deliver much-needed oxygen to your muscles. All of this action means a higher capacity to burn calories—and, in turn, burn fat. You may experience times when you feel like your body is holding on to more water than it needs, and that's okay, too—especially if you're making an effort to change what you're eating. This is when the scale can be deceiving. The scale may show water weight while you've actually lost fat weight.

It's important that you look at your whole person in relation to your weight-loss efforts—not just the constant motion on the scale. Such statements as "I haven't lost a pound this week" reflect reasoning that is destined for failure. Eventually everyone plateaus (see Chapter 6), which is the reality of your body relearning how to metabolize more efficiently and effectively. The more subtle clues of your clothes fitting more loosely, increased energy, and feeling in control are usually a better reality check than what reads on the scale. Often in my practice, between six and eight months after a bypass procedure, patients will come in and lament, "I am stuck—I have not lost a pound in a month." Invariably, they will have lost a pants size in this same time period. But for some patients, going down a clothes size without a remarkable weight loss doesn't count. I have to remind them that this is when a reality check is in order. I then all but guarantee that the weight loss will come again. But until then, the body is unlearning how to maintain weight. In other words, it has to learn to lose as well.

It's also worth pointing out that you'll be gaining lean muscle mass, which, like water, is much heavier than fat. You want as much available water as possible to keep your metabolism in high gear; it will also keep your endurance primed for extended workouts.

Most cells can produce glycogen, which is a stored form of carbohydrate. But the liver and muscle cells store the greatest amounts. After you eat, liver cells obtain the glucose from the blood and convert it to glycogen. Between meals, when blood glucose levels fall, the reaction is reversed, and glucose is released into the blood. This ensures that cells will have a continual supply of glucose to support life. When you take in more carbs than your body can store as glycogen or are needed for normal activities, all that extra glucose becomes fat and is then deposited into your fat cells. The body has an almost unlimited capacity to do this type of conversion, which is why chronic overeating usually leads to obesity.

Tool #5: Eat More Often

We've known for some time now that grazers—those who eat small meals and snacks throughout the day, as opposed to eating three big meals—have an easier time keeping their weight down. I know from what I see among my patients' preoperative habits that eating three square meals a day is a recipe for metabolic disaster. You should eat five meals of between 300 and 500 calories each day. Generally the "lunchtime" and "dinnertime" meals will be on the higher end of the calorie spectrum, and the midmorning and midafternoon meals will be on the lower end—like snacks. This constant eating schedule will help keep your metabolism humming and trigger the body to use good calories for fuel and give up the fat. This explains why someone who cuts back on overall calories may struggle to make excess fat go away. The body senses the reduction in calories, goes into survival mode, and holds tightly onto its fat. When food intake is spread throughout the day, however, this tells your body that it's getting plenty of energy and can let go of the fat! This also has the effect of constantly stretching out that top 10 percent of the stomach, which trains the brain to feel full most or all of the time. There's no time to develop the deep, gnawing hunger that screws up just about any food plan. Just when your fullness signal weakens, it's time to eat again. You've anticipated and met the needs of your brain and body, so there's a significant decrease in cravings, too.

Being famished or, conversely, starving doesn't feel good; the body doesn't like to operate in either of these modes. It much prefers to be fed on a routine basis. Finding that sweet spot in the middle is what eating an ideal combination of food on a regular basis will accomplish. By spacing your meals apart every three to four hours, you'll avoid those energy highs and lows that send your metabolism on a roller coaster. It will keep your metabolism in cruise control and your blood sugar levels stable, which also keeps insulin levels in check. Simply knowing that you get to eat again in a few hours has hidden benefits; you won't have that "last meal" mentality that can lead you to overeat.

Spacing your meals out also helps preserve your internal fat-burning machine: lean muscle mass. If you wait until you're starving, your body will resort to consuming its muscle rather than fat. This has been proven time and time again in clinical studies. One, published in the *British Journal of Nutrition*, showed that weight-loss participants who ate frequent meals preserved considerably more lean muscle tissue than participants who ate fewer daily meals but consumed the same number of calories.

Here's a typical day:

MEAL 1   7 A.M.

MEAL 2   10:30 A.M.

MEAL 3   1 P.M.

MEAL 4   4 P.M.

MEAL 5   6:30 P.M.

(MEAL 6)   (9 P.M.)

The sixth meal is optional, depending on your lifestyle and nutritional needs. You may not want to eat anything within two hours of bedtime, so if you normally go to bed by 10 P.M., you may not need another bite to eat at 9 P.M. and your body can best prepare for sleep if it's not digesting. There are lots of other ways. The basic guideline is to eat every three to four hours to keep your energy levels stable and your metabolism running at high speed.

Though I'd rather you begin to follow your cues of fullness and engage your Portion Police (see next chapter) to know how much you should be eating, I get asked all the time about "how many" calories you should be consuming on a daily basis for weight loss. Most women need a daily average of 1,500 to 1,800 calories; men need 1,600 to 2,200 calories because they have more muscle mass to maintain. Those numbers can change, though, depending on activity levels, body size, and body type. To lose one pound of fat you have to burn 3,500 more calories than you consume. For example, if you burned 500 more calories per day for a total of seven days, by the end of the week you'd have burned enough energy to lose one pound. Five hundred calories may seem like a lot, but not when you consider that you can create that deficit just by cutting 250 calories out of your intake (for example, by swapping out your regular sodas for non-calorie drinks) and upping your activity level (going for a brisk, 30-minute walk).

So don't worry about counting calories. It's virtually impossible to know exactly how many calories you're consuming and what your body is burning anyway. I will encourage you to keep a food journal (see Tool #8), but the purpose of a food journal is not to tabulate calories; it's to keep you mindful of what and how much you're eating throughout the day. If you find yourself popping M&M'S at the office in between meals, and stopping for a mochaccino on your way to pick up the kids, those additional calories will add up. And you'll see them in your journal without having to write down their caloric content.

> Bodybuilders have very little fat because their bodies have been tricked into thinking they do not need to hold on to any fat. How is this possible? They eat around the clock, waking at 2 A.M. for a protein shake and then at 5 A.M. for an egg-white omelet. This constant intake of the right foods is critical to the process of releasing fat. This also explains why super-low-calorie diets backfire.

Tool #6: Choose Your "Supplements" Wisely

No, I'm not referring to vitamin supplements. I'm referring to what I call nonfood foods—the ubiquitous energy bars and drinks. They get sold like candy, but they're marketed as blasts of energy, meal replacements, and on-the-go snacks. I know you'll use them, and that is not a bad thing if they are part of your overall plan. But you need to know *how* to use them so they don't spoil your weight-loss journey. These bars are not created equal; two different "supplements" can have massively different effects on the body. I've had patients gain 15 pounds in a few months just by "adding in a couple of bars a day that my trainer suggested." Why they are taking advice from someone who is treating their nutrition like that of a bodybuilder is beyond me. Eating 400-calorie bars twice a day for a few months really adds up!

First, your food should do something for you. I don't have to spend time telling you to eat whole, real foods. It's what your body wants and craves. Don't you think it stands to reason that most of your diet should consist of what I consider to be real food? The more natural or unmodified a form it is in, the better it is for you. But when we start entertaining the idea of eating supplements in addition to or in place of our meals, that's where things get tricky. You may find yourself eating these supplements in addition to meals, so you're consuming additional calories that you don't need. You may also find that you'll gravitate toward these calorie-dense supplements when all you really need is a calorie-neutral glass of water. Many of these supplements are sold as a way to improve your body's function in life (after all, that word *energy* is a loaded term these days), but usually they are packing on extra calories that will appear on your waistline.

So how do you use these supplements appropriately? As the term implies, they should supplement what you need in your diet. For example, you know I'm a huge advocate of eating five to six meals a day. If you cannot create five to six meals, then I'd prefer that you have a supplemental drink or bar rather than skip a meal. Remember, your body needs a constant supply of resources to burn. Another great way to use supplements it to fulfill a need not met by your meals. If you find it hard to get your daily fill of fiber into your meals, for instance, then grab a fiber-rich supplement to balance that out. If you don't eat enough fruits and veggies, you may need a supplement rich in phytonutrients (you'll know it because the supplement will likely be marketed as providing a certain number of fruits and/or vegetables per serving). If you really are working to increase lean muscle mass, maybe you do need to supplement the amount of protein in your diet. If you want to more consciously limit meal size and encourage fullness, maybe you do need a filling premeal supplement (see Tool #7).

Once again, my basic rules of food intake still apply. Look for bars and drinks that have relatively minimal ingredients, and ingredients you recognize (not a chemistry set!). Watch out for the density of saturated and trans fats, limit sodium, and try and get at least a little bit of protein and fiber. Many supplements are no more than glorified candy bars with photos of bodybuilders on the wrapper—who, by the way, did not get those bodies by eating those bars.

Tool #7: Full Planning

Think of meals as what you plan to eat; they are intentional, and the best time to plan a meal is when you're full. Snacks are what you casually put into your body; they are "whatever is around when you get hungry." Just by planning your foods—the what and when of your eating, the better you will do. And by eliminating spontaneous snacking—or impulse eating—you will better control your weight and nutrition. Remember, a meal is what you plan. A snack is what you grab. I like meals; I don't like snacks. Now, if you're eating five to six meals per day—when are you finding time to snack? Following are some mini-tools for planning your meals successfully and maximizing their fullness effect.

The Premeal Trick: Preload the two biggest meals of your day, which for many are lunch and dinner, with a bulky snack to prompt the Full effect. The science of volumetrics is clearly summed up by recalling Mom's request not to eat anything before dinner because you risked ruining your appetite. She knew that if you had a cookie or ice cream cone or granola bar 30 minutes before dinner, you would not be as hungry. So use that to your advantage by eating something bulky. I like denser foodstuffs with a notable amount of fiber, some protein, and foods that actually need to be chewed to get down. By eating these a half hour before meals— and preferably with a glass of water—you are capitalizing on the hormonal and neurological advantage of the stomach stretch that brings about a feeling of fullness. (Hypothalamus, remember?) A question you might be asking: Can you really eat a midmorning snack, a premeal snack before lunch, an afternoon snack, and a premeal snack before dinner and still control your overall calorie intake for the day? Yes, you can . . . so long as you're choosy about which snacks you eat and how you plan your day in accordance to your body's nutritional needs. Keep in mind that not every day needs to be exactly the same. On some days, your body may want a bigger lunch and a lighter load in the morning. On other days, you'll find that your hunger turns on in the afternoon, perhaps because you worked out at lunchtime, and you'll need to have a decent midafternoon snack and you'll need to preload your dinner with a bowl of cereal. Go with what your body demands but use common sense in deciding what to fill it with; I know you can do this!

Here's a list of premeal snack ideas to get you started, organized from most chewy to least chewy (note that cheeses, breads, and cereals will be higher in calories whereas fruits and veggies will be lower in calories). A general rule to follow is to choose snacks that contain 5 to 14 grams of protein and don't exceed about 200 calories per serving; for additional snack ideas see Appendix D:

- Large supplement bar (look for one that contains at least 3 to 5 grams of fiber)
- Leafy green salad with raw veggies (carrots, celery, bell peppers, mushrooms)
- Small bowl of high-fiber cereal
- 1 to 2 cups of raw vegetables (carrots, broccoli, celery, cauliflower) dipped in 2 tablespoons hummus, low-fat ranch dressing, or salsa
- 1 slice of whole-grain toast with nut butter
- ½ 100% whole-wheat English muffin with 2 tablespoons hummus
- ½ whole-wheat pita and 1 ounce tuna
- 1 ounce beef jerky

- 1 small apple, sliced, with thin slices of cheese

- 1 whole fruit (apple, orange, slices of pineapple, banana, nectarine, peach)

- 1 cup natural popcorn

- A handful of raw nuts

- 1 cup Greek-style nonfat or low-fat yogurt with a sprinkle of 2 tablespoons flaxseed on top

- 2 hard-boiled eggs

- ¾ cup cottage cheese topped with fruit or fruit spread

- 1 cup minestrone or tomato soup (according to research at Penn State University, after participants in a study consumed a vegetable-based, nondairy soup as an appetizer at lunchtime, they ate 20 percent fewer calories than people who skipped the soup)

- Glass of low-fat or nonfat milk (soy, rice, or almond milk is also fine)

Break the Fast, Boost Metabolism: About 40 percent of adults skip breakfast at least four times a week. Although skipping breakfast may seem like a good way to eliminate calories, breakfast skippers tend to be fatter than breakfast eaters. But when people eat a larger-than-normal breakfast, they end up eating almost 100 fewer calories by the end of the day, an amount that can curb creeping obesity. Hence, eating breakfast is one strategy that makes a big difference in weight management (to say nothing of performance at work and in daily activities).

In my practice, one of the hardest things to teach those who are compulsive dieters is that it's important to eat throughout the day. Many are so used to skipping meals to save calories that they are guilt-ridden by the idea of actually eating a prepared breakfast. Every day. In our rushed lives this is the easiest meal to miss and it's a common misconception that cereal companies, for example, are trying to trick us into eating breakfast to sell more boxes of cereal. I am not always an advocate of the breakfast cereal revolution, but cereal companies do have one fact in their favor: breakfast is the most important meal of the day.

Aim to eat breakfast within an hour of rising. After a night's sleep, you need to jump-start your metabolism as soon as possible and bring your blood sugar level back up. Eating breakfast will help you regulate your caloric intake throughout the day and keep your metabolism in cruise control. You won't find yourself craving as many high-calorie, sugary foods later in the day, or eating everything in the house when you get home in the evening.

Your breakfasts should include a balance of quality carbohydrates, protein, and healthy fats. Avoid processed goods such as packaged breakfast bars and Pop-Tarts, which tend to be high in sugar and unhealthy fat. A veggie egg scramble, bowl of hot oatmeal with chopped walnuts, or a fast and easy bowl of cold cereal can do the trick. Pick cereals with at least 3 grams of fiber and fewer than 10 grams of sugar. If you choose a cereal on the sweet or heavy side, mix it with other, lighter cereals. Granola, for example, is typically dense in calories due to its sugar and fat content. Rather than eating a whole bowl of regular granola, sprinkle it on top of a lighter cereal or a bowl of yogurt for an added crunch.

Scheduled Setup: When you don't have a plan for what you're going to eat for dinner by the time you're hungry for it, guess what? That's when it's far too easy to resort to the cheap thrills of fast food and takeout that's low on the nutrient and full meters. Find a day when you can map out a week's worth of meals; for many, Sunday works well. Or pick two days during the week when you can plan about three days' worth of meals if a week is too overwhelming. Make your grocery store list and be choosy about what you buy so you can match your planned menu, including meals you'll make at home and those you'll take with you to work or while on the go. When you make your market run, be sure to have a full stomach prior to stepping out! We all know that shopping while hungry can have unintended consequences. You'll arrive home with loads of food products you never planned on purchasing.

Prepare for Your Environments: The power of planning cannot be overstated. You're always smarter when you're thinking ahead. This allows you to reduce temptation in the heat of the (unplanned) moment. And that temptation, my friends, can also come in the form of friends! When it comes to food, all of us have been sabotaged unintentionally. Researchers like to call this behavior "peer-induced overeating," but we all know what this refers to: being in the company of friends and eating far more than we would have eaten alone. As the number of your dining comrades increases, so does your caloric intake. One study in particular found that eating with eight others can motivate you to consume nearly twice the number of calories you would when alone.

And the heavier your friends, the heavier you're likely to be. According to scientists at Harvard University and the University of San Diego, your risk of becoming overweight skyrockets if you have heavy friends. Hence the headline recently in the media that said something along the lines of "Your friends can make you fat." How is this possible? The simple answer is that it happens as a result of shared behavior. When you've got friends who are overweight, you're not likely to commune over a hike in the hills or an aerobics class; chances are you'll find yourself in an environment conducive to eating and remaining sedentary.

There are people who will always want you to indulge with them. Friendships in general tend to be nurtured in potentially dangerous settings for a waistline, such as at bars and restaurants where there's a lethal mix of alcohol, gab, and mindless gobbling. Don't get me wrong: there's absolutely nothing wrong with mingling with friends in these settings. The key is to be aware of this environment and make use of your tools regardless. My patients have to be especially mindful of their tool (that is, their new anatomy) or they risk getting sick if they eat too much. They can't indulge like they used to, and some of them have to mourn the loss of being able to sit down and pack a huge meal into their bodies. Likewise, you may also have to mourn the loss of habitually eating gigantic meals with friends. It's virtually impossible to avoid all settings that can hinder your success, but it's not impossible to *control* them as best you can. That control ideally should start before you even enter the hazardous setting.

Think about your potential weak spots and vulnerabilities prior to stepping into a "hot zone" of calories and peer pressure. This may be a good time to call on your cheats (again, more on this in Chapter 6.) You don't have to dump your friends; you just have to shift how you let them influence your own personal choices.

Remember, too, that these environments can disrupt your good intentions to stay attuned to your hunger signals. The sight, smell, and talk of food (especially in the company of our friends, no less), will trigger real metabolic signals of hunger even when our stomach is full and in no physical need for food. This helps explain why proximity to fast-food outlets has been linked with weight gain and obesity.

And it gets worse. Subliminal messages abound that can stir up unwarranted feelings of hunger. Ironically, some of these are intended to inspire weight loss. People exposed to posters touting the benefits of *exercise* were found in one study to eat 54 percent more calories than those exposed to posters without a workout theme. Additionally, and oddly, they wanted to eat after reading words like "active." Even your ambient setting can dictate your hunger. Glaring lights on the one hand, and soft lighting on the other, can both contribute to overeating. The thinking goes that bright lights encourage fast and furious eating, whereas candlelight causes us to excessively linger over our food and continue to eat long past the moment when we should have stopped.

So, the environment in which you put yourself can have a huge impact on your eating habits and the level of your consumption. But given this relentless set of weight-antagonizing factors that can thwart just about anyone, one way to fight back is to employ this next tool.

Tool #8: Keep a Journal

One of the critical elements of my bariatric surgery practice is discerning who is not getting the results they want and why. When patients aren't having the success they expect following surgery, I first revert to reminders about the rules of proper tool use. Are they eating small meals frequently throughout the day? Do they drink enough water? Have they unwittingly started to invite caloric snacks into their day like energy bars and coffee shakes without realizing how much they are really consuming? Then, I am very fast to invoke the influence of my dietitians. I require at least a week of meticulous food logging to get a real-life perspective on what they are doing. There is no better window into one's behaviors and the economics of weight loss than to use a food journal. And the mindfulness that accompanies its use is epic.

Science has also proven that keeping a journal during your weight loss can have profound effects on your success. In fact, maintaining a food diary may double your weight loss, according to a recent study from Kaiser Permanente's Center for Health Research—making it the single most successful weight-loss method of all. The findings, from one of the largest and longest-running weight-loss maintenance trials ever conducted, were published in 2009 in the *American Journal of Preventive Medicine*. Scientists at several clinical-research centers in the United States found that dieters who kept a food diary lost *twice* as much weight as those who didn't. In the six-month study, participants who kept a food journal six or seven days a week lost an average of 18 pounds, compared with an average of 9 pounds lost by those who didn't keep a journal. The study tracked nearly 1,700 overweight or obese men and women across the country that were at least 25 years old.

You can use a journal in a number of ways, from recording your thoughts and feelings, achievements and setbacks, to tracking every single thing you put into your mouth and chronicling your physical activity on a daily or weekly basis. Journaling works because it further holds you accountable to your daily behaviors, while making it easier to identify habits that can lead your weight-loss efforts astray. As you write about your efforts to modify your behavior, you are more likely to follow through on your goals. It appears from this latest study that the simple act of writing down what you eat encourages people to consume fewer calories.

While you may think that you know what you eat, all of us have only a general idea and tend to have selective memory, especially when it comes to the foods that aren't so good for our waistlines and overall health. With a detailed food diary, you can see where those extra calories are coming from and, more important, why you may be gravitating toward them.

If you haven't already started a journal from the exercises you've completed in the previous chapters, I encourage you to do so today! Once again, do not make it complicated. You can use any notebook and start by writing down whatever you put in your mouth. Then you can modify the practice as you go.

Tool #9: Take a Multivitamin

It can be a chore to take a multivitamin on a daily basis, especially if you're someone who hates swallowing pills. Getting all the nutrients you need from food alone, though, can also be a challenge. What's more, the body runs more efficiently (read: optimizes its metabolism) when it has all the raw ingredients with which to work. Luckily there are a lot of multivitamins on the market today from which to choose, including vitamin drops you can add to drinks if you really don't like pills, or chewable vitamins flavored to taste like candy (most of these are geared for children, but there's nothing wrong with taking them as an adult so long as you're getting the amounts you need).

Any nutrition store or health-food market will be able to help you choose a multivitamin. To avoid upsetting your stomach, take your multivitamin with food, and you may want to save your vitamin for lunchtime. This will give you a boost of extra nutrients midday and help prevent that afternoon slump that could have you lumbering up to the coffee bar or hitting the vending machine.

Tool #10: Sleep It Off

A classic, positive side effect that I see routinely in my patients is extra energy. As the weight comes off, the surge of energy descends upon them like a force of nature. And as such, I often hear stories from people who proudly exclaim that they are getting by with so much less sleep. Whereas their sleep was previously disrupted by

Boost your levels of vitamin D. Vitamin D, the sunshine vitamin that we can manufacture in our skin upon exposure to UVB radiation, has gained a lot of attention in recent years. An enormous body of research confirms its role in human health and the fact that we don't get enough of it. There's also a growing consensus that the current recommendations (400 IU per day) are far below what we really need for optimal health. Moreover, a 2009 study at the University of Minnesota in Minneapolis explored the connection between vitamin D deficiency and obesity. When researchers measured people's blood levels of vitamin D at the start of the study and then had them adhere to a low-calorie diet for 11 weeks, they discovered that for each increased nanogram per milliliter of vitamin D, dieters lost an additional half pound. In fact, those who had higher levels of vitamin D tended to lose more abdominal fat. Vitamin D experts are currently decoding vitamin D's positive effects on metabolism and are increasingly understanding the critical role it may play in keeping the body disease-free.

sleep disorders related to their obesity, they now experience deeper, restful sleep and for the first time in a long time, they feel full of life and vitality. I have great recollections of stories from guys cleaning their home's gutters at five in the morning "because they are up and have not been able to do it in some time." Or wives who happily report that they "vacuum constantly"—much to their annoyed family's chagrin. These patients say they have "never had a cleaner house" because they have so much energy . . . until the sleep deprivation catches up to them and their weight-loss efforts.

As nice as this burst of productivity can be, it's tempered by what is typically seen as an early plateau accompanying it. In essence, sacrificing sleep can undermine their weight loss. It doesn't give their body time to recover and heal—especially if they have become more physically active.

There's something to be said for looking "refreshed" upon waking from a good night's sleep or nap and feeling more energized. Sleep medicine has come a long way in the past 20 years, and now it's a highly regarded field of study that continues to uncover surprising insights into the power of sleep in the support of health and even weight loss. Just about every system in the body is affected by the quality and amount of sleep you get at night. Sleep can dictate how much you eat, how fat you become, whether you can fight off infections quickly, and how well you can cope with stress.

A study published in 2005, for instance, looked at 8,000 adults over several years as part of the National Health and Nutrition Examination Survey. Sleeping fewer than seven hours a night corresponded with a greater risk of weight gain and obesity, and the risk increased for every hour of lost sleep. In 2009, the *American Journal of Clinical Nutrition* took a small group of men and measured their food intake across two 48-hour periods, one in which they slept eight hours and another in which they slept only four. After the night of shorter sleep, the men consumed more than 500 extra calories (roughly 22 percent more) than they did after eight hours of sleep. Note: 500 more calories a day equals a pound of fat in just a week! A more recent University of Chicago study had similar findings in both men and women: subjects took in significantly more calories from snacks and carbohydrates after five and a half hours of sleep than after eight and a half hours.

You probably know from your own experience that sleep deprivation can encourage you to overeat, drink too much caffeine, and dodge workouts because you're just too tired. Contrary to what you might think, sleep is not a state of inactivity in which our bodies press the pause button for a few hours. During sleep a lot goes on at the cellular level. Clearly, a night of poor sleep or no sleep won't kill you, but prolonged sleep deprivation can put you at high risk for serious weight gain and the inability to take it off, no matter how hard you try. Laboratory and clinical studies have also proven sleep's sweeping role in our lives. Among the many side effects of poor sleep habits are hypertension, confusion, memory loss, the inability to learn new things, weight gain, obesity, cardiovascular disease, and depression. How is this possible?

First, it helps to understand the concept of circadian rhythms, a natural cycle of biological activity that changes throughout the 24-hour day. This rhythm revolves around our sleep habits and the shifts from daytime to nighttime. A healthy day-night cycle is linked to how our body produces and circulates hormones, including those associated with our eating patterns and those that relate to stress, metabolism, and cellular recovery and renewal. The stress hormone cortisol, for example, should be highest in the morning and progressively decrease throughout the day. It should be at its lowest point after 11 P.M., which is when melatonin levels peak. Melatonin is your body's hormone for signaling sleep, and it typically starts pumping from your pineal gland when it's dark outside. Once released, melatonin has several functions: it downshifts the body's operations, lowers blood pressure, and, in turn, core body temperature. All of this ultimately prepares you for sleep. Higher melatonin levels facilitate deeper sleep, which helps maintain healthy levels of growth hormone, thyroid hormone, and male and female sex hormones. If you've ever had a tough time winding down at night due to stress, you may be secreting too much cortisol, which competes with the sleep-enhancing melatonin.

Sleep is associated with lots of hormones. When you reach deep sleep, which is about a half an hour after you first close your eyes, your pituitary gland at the base of your brain releases high levels of growth hormone (GH). Although GH gets released throughout the night during your sleep cycles, the peak surge is highest just after you fall asleep. Growth hormone is responsible for many tasks in the body beyond stimulating growth and cell reproduction. It also refreshes cells and restores the skin's elasticity, enhances the movement of amino acids through cell membranes, and even helps you to maintain an ideal weight. It does this by telling your cells to switch from using carbs to fat for energy. Without adequate sleep, GH cannot escape the pituitary, which negatively affects your proportions of fat to muscle. And over time, low GH levels are associated with high fat and low, lean muscle.

Most of my patients don't think about their sleep habits as they consider a dramatic measure like surgery to gain control of their weight. Yet sleep is such a noninvasive strategy to weight loss, though it's sometimes not so easy to get. As I explained in Chapter 3, the two digestive hormones that control your feelings of hunger and appetite are ghrelin (your "Go eat" hormone) and leptin (your "I'm full" hormone). Ghrelin gets secreted by the stomach when it's empty and sends a message to your brain that you need to eat. When your stomach is full, fat cells send out the leptin so your brain gets the message that you can stop eating now. One of the most exciting findings revealed in the past decade includes how out of whack these hormones get after insufficient sleep. When people are allowed just four hours of sleep a night for two nights, they experience a 20 percent drop in leptin and an increase in ghrelin. They also have a marked increase (about 24 percent) in hunger and appetite. And they gravitate toward calorie-dense, high-carbohydrate foods such as sweets, salty snacks, and starchy foods. Sleep loss essentially deceives your body into believing it's hungry when it's not, and it also tricks you into craving foods that can sabotage a healthy diet. What's more, because we need sleep to metabolize glucose properly, sleep loss over time can lead to diabetes. Sleep deprivation impairs the body's ability to use insulin, the hormone responsible for maintaining stable blood-sugar levels.

Sleep deprivation is epidemic, and most of us don't get the sleep we really need. On average, we get an hour less sleep per day than we did 40 years ago. I can go on and on about the value of sleep and the role it plays in our lives from both a physical and, let's not forget, psychological standpoint. But that's another book. Everyone has a different sleep need. The "eight-hour" rule is general, because most people do need seven to nine hours, which makes an average of eight. If you feel like a drag after a five-hour night, then clearly you need to get more sleep. Think of the last time you went on vacation and slept like a baby for more hours a night than usual. Whatever you averaged on vacation is probably closer to your daily sleep requirement.

Despite what many people attempt to do, shifting your sleep habits on the weekends to "catch up" can undermine a healthy circadian rhythm. To sleep soundly every night, plan to go to bed and wake up at exactly the same time, seven days a week. Give yourself at least 30 minutes to prepare for sleep by avoiding stimulating activities so your body is in a relaxed state when you slip into bed. Last, limit your caffeine intake after 2 P.M., and try not to drink alcohol within a few hours of bedtime so it can be metabolized rather than disrupt your sleep cycles.

The Full Challenge: Day 4

All of the above tools meet two criteria: (1) they don't feel like a dreaded diet, and (2) they optimize the Full effect. I know that if it's not easy, you won't do it. Or, worse, you'll start and then stop when it feels like a chore. That is what I am fighting against.

In the previous chapter, I helped you to become more mindful of your eating behavior and the steps to digestion that are under your control. And in the next chapter I'll offer up examples of a perfect day's worth of eating, so your challenge for today is to choose one tool—*just one*—from numbers 3 to 10 to apply to your life today. Don't go crazy, and don't try to do a handful all at once. Trying to use too many will likely lead you to falter and then have an excuse to bail out of this program. I will not make it that easy for you. You're not a computer and this is not a computer program. This is a basic way of adapting your habits to a more healthful manner that encourages weight control.

Think simple and focus on progress. Don't set yourself up for failure by making an elaborate plan with 14 steps. If you miss a step, you'll feel like a failure and give up—even though you've accomplished a lot already. Instead, create realistic goals and a specific way to get started, with just one tool. Then, focus on progress even if you find yourself not doing *exactly* what you set out to do. If you manage to cut out soda most days of the week, but slip up over the weekend, don't beat yourself up. You're still drinking fewer liquid calories than you were a week ago. Keep it up, and you'll begin to think of yourself as a nonsoda person— drinking just water will become part of your identity. And going from drinking soda part-time to none at all will be a lot easier than going from full-time to cutting cold turkey.

BARBORA FAGAN

Age: 26, Height: 5'6"
Starting: Weight: 180.4, Size: 12
Final: Weight: 156.2, Size: 8
Total Lost: 24.2 Pounds and 25.75"

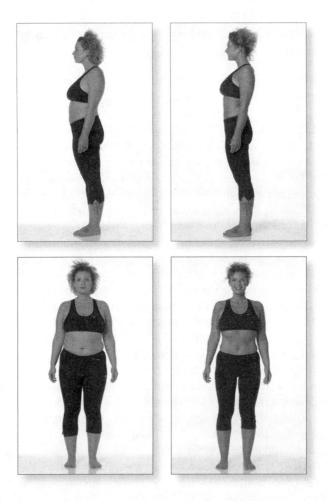

"As a restaurant manager, I'm around food all day. But this program has focused me and I feel so good that it's easy to make a few lifestyle changes using the tools. I'm so thrilled to be thinner than when I got married, and I'm excited to celebrate my fifth anniversary with a new body."

CHAPTER FIVE
DAY 5

YOUR PORTION POLICE

Portion control is so important that I've written an entire chapter on it. It may, in my opinion, be the most important tool people can use—whether they choose a steady diet of crispy bacon, fried chicken, and ice cream; or fruits, nuts, and berries.

While in my second year of surgical residency and newly married, my wife and I decided to eat less fat. A wise idea, as I was packing in pizza, whole-milk lattes, and candy bars while awaiting the constant influx of trauma choppers that would interrupt my sleep. Out of love, my wife began to wean me off of my usual big bowl of ice cream with syrup and malt powder and replaced it with prepared low-fat cakes. But, presented with a low-fat cake, I always ate the whole thing. Serving size: 8! Obviously, my weight did not improve. I was seemingly "eating well" because I wasn't eating fat. But I clearly did not grasp the concept of reasonable portions.

In my bariatric patients' first year after surgery, they become experts at judging how much they should eat. I have taught them to know exactly what six to eight ounces of food looks like, and at their one-year anniversary post-op, when I ask them on a form, "How much do you eat per meal?" the response is nearly unanimous: "Full with six to eight ounces of food." At their second-year anniversary, however, the responses aren't always so uniform. Some patients get cavalier. It's not intentional, but I frequently see that people plateau

113

above where they want to be or gain back some weight. And, almost always, this is the result of forgetting how much to eat at a given meal. When asked, they may say, "I eat the fajitas until I am full— I have no idea how much I eat." I remind them that a year ago they knew *exactly* how much they ate.

This chapter guides you through understanding how much to eat. For you, the rules will be different than those of my patients, but based on the same physiological facts. Even though I spent Chapter 3 describing how we are wired to sense fullness, the concept of eating until you are full is a recipe for disaster if you're constantly courting fullness. It takes experience and a great deal of self-awareness to reach the point where you can rely on feelings of fullness to push away from the table. We must start with visual cues that will then help you to tune into your physiological cues. Moreover, without a consideration for volume, it's easy to push past feelings of fullness and elevate your tolerance for more food than you need. Have you ever had an illness that caused you to lose your appetite? Then when the illness passes, you seem able to eat less? This is because your stomach has grown used to eating less and seems to "have shrunk." Although the "shrinking part" isn't real, you have taught your body to physically be satisfied with less.

Taking the guesswork out of how much you should eat is actually simple. Let me walk you through this step by step.

Mind Before Matter

Before eating anything (meal or snack), get your journal out and keep track of the answers to the following two questions:

1. How hungry am I? (use a scale of 1 to 10, 1 being "uncomfortably starving" and 10 being "uncomfortably overstuffed"; you are "comfortably full" at 5).

2. Is my desire for food being triggered by feelings such as stress or boredom?

This second question often can be difficult to answer. Be honest, though, even if it entails confronting feelings you may not want to deal with. We all tend to think of (and seek out) food when we are stressed, bored, tired, frustrated, anxious, sad, mad, moody, and so on. It's human nature to have our emotions connected to our desire to eat. You may want to ask yourself the following specific questions:

I am feeling: _____.

I want to eat because: _____.

I need to eat because: _____.

If I eat, I will feel: _____.

The last time I ate was at (give time): _____.

The last things I ate were: _____.

I realize that you may not be actively journaling—against my good advice! But, at least take a few moments to consider these specific questions. Think about keeping them on a card in your purse or wallet. Make this inquiry a part of the prelude to every meal or occasion to eat.

The goal of pausing before eating to write down these thoughts is to begin a practice of mindful eating (see Tool #2). Though I'm encouraging you to take your time eating so you can maximize the effect of the fullness sensors in your brain and avoid overriding them, there's another reason to slow down at your next meal. Eating slowly reinforces this mindful effect. According to a study involving college women and large plates of pasta, those instructed to eat quickly consumed an average of 646 calories in nine minutes. When these same women were told to chew 15 to 20 times per bite, they ate 579 calories in 29 minutes and reported feeling full an hour later. That can amount to a huge difference over time.

Mindful eating is not something I made up; it's actually a movement that now has lots of research to back up how beneficial it can be on long-term weight loss. In basic terms, mindfulness is simply a return to paying attention. When we pay attention to our food—and I mean really pay attention with all of our senses—we begin to notice many wonderful aspects of the food, and we become aware of how much we're putting into our bodies.

The main objectives of mindful eating include: learning to make better choices at the start or toward the end of a meal based on your awareness of hunger and "full" cues; learning to identify personal triggers for mindless eating, such as emotions, social pressures, habits, or certain foods; valuing quality over quantity of what you're eating; appreciating the sensual, as well as the nourishing, capacity of food; and feeling deep gratitude that may come from appreciating and experiencing food.

As I've been hinting at since the beginning of this book, food is not necessarily the problem when it comes to weight control. Nor does the problem stem from your fat cells, stomach, or intestines. The crux of the problem lies in the mind—in our lack of awareness of the messages coming in from our body, from our very cells, and from our heart. Mindful eating helps us learn to hear what our body is telling us about hunger and fullness. It helps us become aware of who in the body/heart/mind complex is hungry, and how and what will best nourish it.

Much of mindful eating has been based on the field of meditation. As with meditation, mindful eating helps us to focus our attention on the present moment rather than the past or future. Taking this approach ultimately helps us to disconnect from habits and behaviors that may sabotage our goals and wishes. For example, if you've ever found yourself gorging on a meal that's only marginally satisfying and leaves you feeling overstuffed, guilty, and low on energy (and you may not even remember the act of eating itself), then you know what it means to fall victim to a habitual binge with few rewards. Eating mindfully means paying attention to what you're doing rather than chowing down absentmindedly while doing something else such as watching television. It also means passing up that gargantuan tub of popcorn at the movies that costs only a dollar more than the small version.

Simple activities can inspire you to eat less and think more. Over a ten-year period, middle-aged people who practiced yoga gained less weight than those who didn't practice yoga. Researchers who noted this difference speculate that yogis bring the mindfulness they learn in class to the table with them and end up consuming fewer calories.

With mindful eating, it's possible to discover a far more satisfying relationship with food, and even with ourselves, by slowing down, enjoying every bite, and noticing how we are feeling—in our mind, heart, and stomach. It's also possible to control what and how much we are eating without iron willpower. And when we succeed at mindful eating, the nourishment we then experience is not just physical; it's deeply emotional, and for some, spiritual as well. If you've never tried to eat mindfully, it may sound impossible to take only a few bites of, say, chocolate and be fully satisfied. But you'd be surprised by how powerful mindful eating can be. It's true that after four or five bites, your taste buds lose their sensitivity to the chemicals in a particular food that make it taste good. And it's "taste-specific satiety" that explains why the first bites of chocolate taste better than later ones and why, when you cannot manage another bite of steak, you have plenty of enthusiasm for ice cream. Once you recognize that you're losing the pleasure of a certain taste, it's easier to stop. Mindful eating takes the power away from food and places that power in your hands. Being more aware is much easier to do than relying on willpower, don't you think?

Over the past 25 years, mindfulness practices in general have been shown to have a positive impact on many areas of psychological and physical health, including stress, depression, anxiety, chronic pain, and heart disease. More recently, evidence is building that validates the benefits of mindful eating for treatment of obesity as well as binge eating disorders. The benefits of mindful eating are not restricted to physical and emotional health improvements. They can also impact one's entire life, through a greater sense of balance and well-being.

When you feel in control, you no longer have to live in fear of your next meal. You can rely on your natural cues of fullness and respond to their messages automatically. This has the added advantage of giving you control of your thoughts. Many of my patients lament the constant and intrusive bombardment of thoughts about food. *Am I hungry? Should I eat? Will this be good for me? Will I gain another pound? Should I avoid eating this? Will this make me fatter? Can I avoid thinking about food for 20 minutes?*

Don't underestimate the power of journaling for keeping you mindful. As I outlined in the previous chapter, tracking food and activity is a proven way to identify your habits, trigger foods, and underlying emotions that play a role in your eating patterns. If we add the task of tracking levels of fullness, emotions, and feelings to our journaling, I bet we can enhance the probability of success. Anecdotal evidence from my own practice has shown this to be true. In addition, entering this information into your journal will be a powerful motivator to help keep you working toward your goals.

Pop Quiz: Do you know how to practice mindful eating? Try the following at your next opportunity:

Take a sip of hot tea or coffee with full attention. Don't do anything else but drink (no television, talking, e-mail checking, and so on) and think about the flavor and heat of the drink.

Sit down at a table with a book and a snack. Read one page and then put the book down, take a couple bites of your snack, and think about what you just read as you enjoy the taste sensations in your mouth. Do not return to reading until a few seconds after you have finished swallowing.

Eat a meal alone and in silence. Make sure it takes at least 20 minutes for you to polish off the plate. For entertainment, you can look out a window or reflect on photos nearby, but do not access the television, Internet, reading material, or even another human being. Just you and your meal. That's it!

Single Serving

The most nutritious meal can be toxic if you don't know when to say, "I've had enough." Yes, even a perfect meal—balanced complex carbohydrates, fats, and proteins derived from organic ingredients and prepared with love in your own kitchen—is harmful to your waistline if you're eating a bushel of it!

You get one plate of food. You can follow whatever dietary guidelines you wish, though I highly recommend that you use at least one of the tools described in the previous chapter about which types of foods to favor. See if you can build your meals around lean proteins and vegetables. For example, try aiming for a plate that's one-third protein, one-half vegetables, and the rest a small portion of a starch or grain. In terms of servings, that amounts to one serving of protein, two servings of vegetables (or one serving of vegetables and one serving fruit), and one small serving of starches or grains.

If it helps, use a 7-inch plate or 2-cup bowl rather than the more common 9-inch plate and deep-dish bowl.

Dish Out Your Portion

Decide how much you are going to eat *before your first bite* and place it all on your plate. There are two ways to go about this: (1) you can use your own judgment for serving yourself a smart portion, or (2) buy eight-ounce food-storage containers and fill those first. Does your meal fit into an eight-ounce container? If not, remove some food until the contents fit (with a sealed top). If this truly doesn't represent enough food for you, then it's okay to start with 12-ounce containers and downsize later. Then assemble the food on a plate. Follow this routine for two weeks or until you can

119

determine the proper amount of food without the container. Even when you no longer need to use the container, lay the empty container beside your plate to stay visually tuned into your portions. And if you do decide to drop the container tool entirely from your meals, you may find that your portions begin to increase in size—without your really knowing it at first. So it helps to check back with your container comparison on a frequent basis. If you start feeling that you are overstuffed after meals or your weight loss stalls or perhaps your weight increases, you'll know it's time to bring that container out again for help in creating your ideal serving.

Seeing Full vs. Feeling Full: There's a reason why we're using visual cues to help you tune into your physiological cues. You are learning about the volume that makes you feel full. And, when looked at from this visual and mindful perspective, you may be amazed that less is enough. Virtually everyone puts what they think is a "serving" on their plate before eating—then eats the whole "serving" (or just about). Only by being better able to gauge what a true serving is will you be able to make the appropriate changes.

As you know, I am really trying to keep it simple and keep you out of the clutches of those who want you to be measuring and weighing what you take in. We all know how poorly that has turned out for us. But, at the same time, I cannot allow you to eat huge volumes (even if you're eating the "right stuff"), so you need to start somewhere. The only way to make progress toward an intelligent dietary regimen is to start to address the issue of finding an acceptable volume for you.

Don't panic the first time you measure out your meal and worry that it won't be enough or that you're eating the wrong foods. You do not have to be perfect all of the time. Boring. Instead, I want you to strive for about 90 percent "really good." If you're not full I'll let you add more food once you check in with your sense of fullness. Make it a goal to eat your meal slowly. Rather than wolfing down everything within minutes, see if you can lengthen the time it takes for you to consume your meal. Then, you'll check in.

Check In at 20 Minutes

About 20 to 30 minutes after your meal—when the physical, nervous, and hormonal elements of fullness are reaching their peak—ask yourself how you feel. On that scale of 1 to 10, how full are you? Record your answers in your journal. Here are my parameters:

"**1 to 3: I am still hungry.**" Either you didn't eat enough, didn't actively search out the foods that make you feel more full, such as those rich in protein and fiber, or you didn't wait long enough before you assessed fullness. It takes at least a full 20 to 30 minutes for your brain to register fullness. Has it been that long? If you determine that you, in fact, didn't eat enough to satisfy your body's needs, then this may mean actively measuring out your food for a while to make sure you know what amounts will give you a true sense of fullness. For example, if you're starting with 8 ounces and it takes 12 ounces to feel full, that's important to know. But you have to be sure you're actively pursuing an ideal amount of food for your body and not fooling yourself.

Daily Servings and Serving Sizes

Protein: There are various types of proteins to consider when planning your meals and snacks. These include animal protein, vegetable protein, dairy, legumes, and nuts. Make sure to include one serving of animal or vegetable protein in every meal or two to three servings of dairy or legumes. Feel free to mix and match. Generally, I would recommend that cheese, milk, yogurt, nuts and nut butters be saved for snacks or used as part of a mix of proteins for a meal. If choosing animal proteins, make sure to select lean meats most of the time. Refer to pages 84–85 for examples of lean and medium-to high-fat proteins. Serving sizes:

- *Animal and vegetable protein:* 3 to 5 ounces cooked weight, or the size of a deck of cards; for those with a larger appetite, start with a double deck of cards

- *Dairy:* 1 cup yogurt or milk, 1 ounce cheese
- *Legumes:* 1 cup cooked peas or beans
- *Nuts and nut butters:* 1 ounce nuts, 2 tablespoons nut butters

Vegetables: Vegetables are unlimited and should be eaten at will, but aim to have at least 4 servings of cooked or raw vegetables per day. If you cut up raw vegetables and keep them on hand, it makes a convenient snack that will encourage you to grab these when you're hungry. You can easily add vegetables to each meal, including breakfast and snacks. Consider adding vegetables to your eggs. Remember, starchy vegetables, such as potatoes, sweet potatoes, and corn, are considered in the "Grain/Starch" food group and not as vegetables. Serving sizes:

- *Raw or cooked veggies:* ½ cup
- *Vegetable juice:* ½ cup
- *Leafy raw vegetables*: 1 cup

Fruit: Most men and active women should eat at least 2 servings of fruit every day. Serving size:

- *Large fruits:* 1 whole piece about the size of a tennis ball
- *Small fruits:* 1 cup

Grains/Starch: At a given meal, most adults consume two servings of grains, such as a cup of cooked rice or two slices of bread. While you're trying to lose weight, try to limit to 3 servings of grain/starch per day. Once you reach the weight you want to maintain, the servings can be increased to 5 to 8 servings per day depending on your activity level. The more active you are, the greater the number of servings. Serving size:

- *Bread:* 1 slice
- *Cereal or granola:* 1 ounce
- *English muffin or bagel:* ½ piece
- *Rice, pasta, cereal, or quinoa:* ½ cup, cooked
- *Starchy vegetables:* ½ cup
- *Tortilla:* 1 small

You may need to ask yourself if you have an unrealistic expectation of what fullness is. If you repeatedly need to be stuffed, then that's what you'll crave—the feeling of being stuffed. I'd rather you aim to be adequately full so you're not hungry enough to want to eat. With my patients, I regularly have them assess how full is full enough. When they do this, they find it's always less than what they imagined they would need. On a scale of 1 to 10, I want them to get to a maximum of 6 to 7 of fullness. Remember, you're supposed to be eating again in another three to four hours, so how full do you need to be? Even if you decide to go for more food after 20 minutes, write down where you are on the fullness scale in your journal and record your additional intake.

"5: I am okay; not too full, but not hungry." If you're already at a 5, stop. This is the magic moment. When you realize how much it takes to actually feel adequately full and you don't feel like you're living without, then from that point on, you can make rational decisions about controlling your intake. It's truly magic when you can say, "I'm done with the right amount of food and a good balance of carbs, fat, and protein." Your body will function better, you'll feel better, and you'll control your weight more effectively.

If you're close to a 5 (say, a 4), then add just a little bit more on your plate in the form of lean protein and fibrous vegetables, wait 20 minutes, and reassess. If you find yourself over a 5 (say, a 6 or 7), then you know to cut back a little on your plate.

"8 to 10: I am really full." You've eaten too much food and you probably surpassed your fullness sensation. It may be that you ate too fast because you couldn't employ that 20- to 30-minute rule. By the time your brain got the message that you were full, you had already eaten more. Next time, eat less. Downsize your meal. Experiencing too much fullness can be beneficial: it almost certainly teaches you that your brain is trying to make you think you need more food than you do to be full and happy. It's critical that you know what volume of what foods it takes to eat well and not deny yourself. Give yourself time to feel full. Eat a respectable amount and then wait a half hour to see how you feel.

Factor in Other Variables to Levels of Hunger: Other factors to consider when assessing your body's biological hunger and how much it really needs to sustain its energy include: dehydration, activity level, hormonal fluctuation, and skipping meals. In my practice, I count all of these factors. There is always a key to one's stagnation or lack of progress. And in my experience, a person is never "cursed" to not lose enough. That would be way too convenient an excuse to stop trying! So, like an archaeologist, we have to look at each stratum of what makes up one's life and weight-control efforts. Let's take a look at each of the four "stratum":

- *Dehydration*: It's easy to mistake thirst for hunger, so before serving yourself more food you may want to try drinking an eight-ounce glass of water, wait another ten minutes, and see if your hunger diminishes.

- *Activity level*: The amount of food your body needs may vary. One day you may be active or recovering from an active day and your body needs more energy in the form of more food. Another day you may be sedentary and not needing as much food. Activity levels change daily, and there is no magic portion total that will meet your individual and constantly evolving needs day after day, meal after meal. So view consumption more broadly and allow room for flexibility. At a given meal, you may need more food for whatever reason. Respond to that hunger and take in an extra serving. Remember, you are training your body to feel full with the right amount of food for you. My hope is that you can do away with my baseline rules once you can successfully adopt this way of eating as a lifetime practice.

- *Hormonal fluctuation*: Most women can attest to the fact that hormones affect hunger. The fluctuating hormone levels during a woman's menstrual cycle, peri-menopause, and menopause can dramatically impact how much she feels like eating and even what she craves. You may find, for instance, that you crave fat and sugar or have a harder time controlling your portions during certain times of the month. This is when being especially mindful of the foods you choose is key. Be aware of your eating habits and portion sizes, and be extra cautious about treats. You may even want to store up your cheats (a topic covered in the next chapter) for the days during the week when you know your hormones could be talking to you. Use your journal to chart your hormonal changes. Become more aware of them and how they are affecting your eating habits.

- *Skipping meals*: If you find yourself ravenous at a particular meal, you waited too long to eat. How long has it been? Did you skip breakfast (and if breakfast was just a blended coffee and muffin, that doesn't really count)? When you follow the three- to four-hour guideline, you shouldn't arrive at any meal wanting to eat everything in the kitchen. If it has been a long time, try using the premeal trick: eat a small snack about 30 minutes before your main meal (see previous chapter for details). This will take the edge off your hunger and help you to regulate your portion.

Due to their new stomach dimensions, my patients have a unique experience with portion control soon after surgery. After they're done healing, their new stomach is about two ounces in size, or the size of an egg. Once they reengage in real-life eating, which includes going out to dinner and encountering settings where it's hard to control portions, they can quickly forget that there's an extreme limit to the amount they can eat. They will sit down with an order of shrimp cocktail and forget that their stomach cannot physically accommodate six whole shrimp. If they finish the dish, they will vomit thereafter. And it usually takes three such episodes of overeating and throwing up for them to realize that there's a true, sensible amount of space in their stomach that will allow them to eat safely, comfortably, and effectively for weight loss.

You're not much different. Although you're working with much more space in your stomach, you too have limits. Once you're aware of how you should court fullness and need an acceptable amount to be comfortably full, only then can you get on with your life. It may be un-American to eat a reasonably sized meal that makes us comfortably full given what we're in front of most of the time, but it's still the right way to eat. To underscore how outrageous our portions have gotten, consider this: I once was in Florence, Italy, and came across a gelato shop that sold the cold confection in four sizes—small (1 scoop), medium (2 scoops), large (3 scoops), and the "American," which had a whopping 16 scoops! The Italians knew that we Americans like to "get full" on our indulgences.

Bring Reality to Restaurants

Do not get tricked into overindulgence by the outrageous serving sizes at most restaurants. You can still use your food containers to assess portion size even when you go out. Bring your food container with you to make your measurement, and then pack up the extra food in that container to take home. Or ask for a doggie bag as soon as your food arrives so you can separate the food you're going to eat at the restaurant from the portion you'll take home. Alternatively, share entrées with your dining companions or order an appetizer and eat it as an entrée. In many restaurants, an appetizer can be the perfect portion for a single serving. Or you can do what my mom does: she actually "contaminates" her extra food by putting it onto a separate plate and salting it to death. (I know it seems wasteful, but work with me here. I'll explain its effectiveness later.) She does this with huge dessert servings, too.

Not All Salads Are Created Equal

The word *salad* can be quite deceiving. Some restaurants will serve bowls of greens that contain more calories and fat than other dishes on the menu that sound obviously heavy, such as burgers and fries. Salads have long been considered "diet foods," but they can spoil the best weight-loss plans. The reasons might surprise you. It's not only that salads may be loaded down with calorie-heavy ingredients such as bacon bits, cheese, croutons, nuts, dried fruit, avocado, and creamy dressings; they can also give you the *illusion* that you're eating well when you're not. This warped misperception can then make you feel entitled to indulge in something else—or eat twice as much of a heavy salad than if you had chosen a reasonably sized sandwich and small side salad.

If you're the type who always orders salads, you may be inadvertently shooting yourself in the foot. In other words, if you don't allow yourself to vary your meals, you may find your caloric intake increasing over time as you slowly but surely find ways to sneak appetizing breaks from the monotony. I see this all the time among patients who unwittingly waver from their tools and personal plans because they crave more variety. But rather than applying those same tools and sense of portion control to other options, they let themselves loose—and lose sight of how much they are eating. For example, you may think you're "being good" when you order the split pea soup and spinach salad, but then forget any self-control over the bread basket or take the lion's share of the artichoke dip that is meant for the whole table.

What's more, studies have shown that seeing the word *salad* on a menu can have some unintended psychological consequences.

The word *salad* can make you choose the least healthy item on a menu even if you'd normally practice self-restraint and control. In an alarming study at Duke University, people were presented with one menu that offered a baked potato with butter, chicken nuggets, or French fries. Another menu listed the same items but added a side salad. When the side of greens was an option, nearly three times as many people ordered the fries. Even people who said they typically watched what they ate found themselves switching from the potato (which was considered the healthiest of the items on the first menu) to the fries. The researchers suggested that the mere option of eating healthy made the diners feel as if they had already achieved a goal, and could thus reward themselves for that by choosing an indulgent option.

Salads can be very filling when they include ingredients that speak to your sense of fullness. Bulky, fibrous greens; kale; spinach; and raw veggies such as celery, bell peppers, and mushrooms will hit your full sensors quickly. They don't work as well when they are loaded down with ingredients that add crunch, sweetness, and sometimes saltiness. You can fool yourself into thinking you're eating a 200-calorie salad when in reality, it adds up to more like 600 calories (not to mention all the extra sides you nibble on because you do, in fact, believe you're eating just 200 calories with a little extra here and there). Looks, and sometimes tastes, can be deceiving at the salad bar. Even if you choose the olive oil–based dressing, get it on the side so you can decide how many 120-calorie tablespoons you really want. It doesn't take much.

Ask for What You Want

It's okay to make special requests in restaurants. It's not about what you ask for, but how you ask. Don't be afraid to say no butter added, dressing on the side, baked not fried, please use cooking spray not oil, dry toast, omelets with egg whites, turkey bacon rather than real bacon, light dressing, sub out starches (rice, bread) for extra veggies or fruit, steamed without the sauce, and so on. You'll be surprised by how willing chefs are to make it exactly as

Watch out for foods labeled as "diet" or are thought to be "diet-friendly." Salads can do more harm than a double-bacon cheeseburger in some cases. Portion-controlled snack bags can also lead people astray as they disempower your self-control quite subconsciously. A study out of the Netherlands found that when people were given the option of two large bags of chips or nine snack-size bags, 59 percent of the participants chose the smaller bags. The problem: those who chose the smaller bags ate twice as much as the people who opted for the large bags. The lesson: smaller doesn't always mean less when it comes to total consumption. You have to keep your portion-control thinking cap on at all times.

you like it, and help you find healthier substitutions. And you can always joke, like my wife does every time, by saying something like, "I'm sorry I'm such a pain, but I'm a pretty good tipper!"

Worried about venturing to a new restaurant where you're unfamiliar with the menu? The Internet can help you out. You can usually view the restaurant's menu online. This is a smart move as it will further remove the impulsivity from going out to eat. If you arrive at the restaurant already knowing what to eat and avoid, you've started with an appropriate level of mindfulness. Impulse orders are often what get us in trouble. And remember that most meals served in restaurants today are pumped up with excessive calories and cheap carbohydrates to add volume.

Remember, matching the visual cues with the physiological cues of fullness is our ultimate goal. Once you gain a clear understanding of reasonable portion size, you won't have to second-guess yourself or perpetually eat more than your body really needs. Becoming a master of portion control takes practice, but I trust you will eventually have your own personal aha moment when your brain says you've had enough. The sensation of being full requires no explanation. Like love and hate, the word *full* defines itself. And the ability to be full is in all of us.

The Full Challenge: Day 5

Using the portion information you've learned in this chapter and the food choice discussions from the previous chapter, your Day 5 challenge is to learn how to structure the perfect meal. I realize that this can feel terrifying at first, but it doesn't have to be. Simply sit down and come up with 10 snack ideas and 10 meal ideas that follow the basics I've outlined, and then incorporate these into your life—starting today. If you would prefer to skip this personalizing step and simply start incorporating healthier meals, I've provided 30 days of meal ideas in Appendix C and some snack ideas in Appendix D. Why wait to start eating healthier? Once you learn the ropes to creating or assembling the perfect meal, it will become automatic and effortless. And that's the whole point.

DAYON THOMAS

Age: 36, Height: 5'9"
Starting: Weight: 243.4, Size: 38"
Final: Weight: 224.6, Size: 36"
Total Lost: 18.8 Pounds and 14.25"

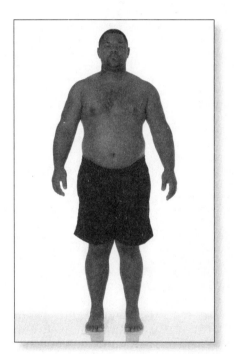 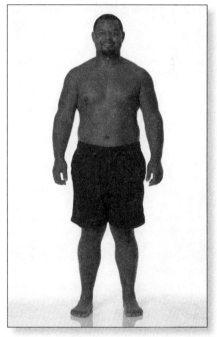

"As a former semi-pro football player, I used to be in good shape. After two kids, my wife lost her pregnancy weight but I still kept my 'sympathy' weight. Within two weeks of the program, I noticed a big difference in my energy, and my stomach had shrunk. The weight has been coming off everywhere—midsection, face, neck—and my chest and arms are more defined."

CHAPTER SIX

YOUR CHEAT AND PLATEAU PRESCRIPTION

I once had a patient who could not stop cheating. She had to have chocolate (especially Hershey's Kisses) daily. After losing 140 pounds from gastric bypass, she was working her way up again—30 pounds regained. She knew that with each indulgence, she was destroying what she had worked so hard to achieve. Every indulgence in her chocolate passion was another step toward climbing into the larger-sized pants that she had abandoned on the way down. Chocolate was running and ruining her life.

I fixed this problem in a very simple way. I told her that I was thrilled that she had discovered her vice and I wanted her to keep eating it. But I wanted her to have more control. I gave her a chocolate budget of a one-pound bag of Kisses per week. She could eat them in any fashion she wanted—all at once, ten per day, whatever. Every Monday she got a new bag. I told her to come back in two weeks for a checkup.

Strangely, when she had permission to eat chocolate—when it was no longer taboo but "prescribed" by her doctor—it ceased to be a big draw. She actually had a difficult time eating all of the chocolate in a week. Then, I told her that I wanted her to eat some chocolate three times per week and to measure it out and only have one sensible serving. However, she got to decide what that serving looked like. When she came in two weeks later, she felt that this was easy. She ate a paper cup full of chocolate chips three times per week and felt totally in control. Her weight started coming down again, and she no longer felt like a failure.

I have seen the same thing with mochas, Doritos, popcorn, margaritas, Coke, cookies, Slurpees . . . you name it. We have *all* experienced the cycle of indulgent eating. It is miserable. We think that we've screwed it all up and have no control. We then allow ourselves to cheat like crazy. The cure I've discovered is to allow my patients to be themselves—with all of their desires and passions. And that's why I developed cheat prescriptions.

This chapter gives you a specific prescription for managing those foods you find it hard to resist—your cheats. I'll take you through creating and managing your own food cheats no matter what those are. I'll even include cheats for indulgences other than food, such as having days off from exercise (the exercise component is a topic saved for the next chapter, but I'll talk about it within the context of cheating, which speaks to those already accustomed to a routine). I'll also give you troubleshooting tactics for handling the unexpected, such as being confronted with a box of cookies or doughnuts at work when they haven't been factored into your cheat Rx. Last, I'll help you break through plateaus when your weight loss stagnates.

Why Cheat?

Cheating sounds bad, but it doesn't have to be. Cheat plans counterbalance the threat posed by denying yourself something you really want. Cheat plans allow you to indulge without ruining everything. When we try to be perfect, we end up failing because we set too high a standard. Then, since we believe we wrecked everything, we overindulge—and feel guilty.

We all need permission to have a carbohydrate hangover—the day after an indulgent carb-rich day for which you may physically feel a little off. This is good because it helps you get back on track. It can help you in more ways than you can imagine, actually. According to a University of Michigan study, when dieters satisfied a craving in a small portion- and calorie-controlled way, they subsequently did a better job of resisting temptation.

And that's exactly the goal of my cheat prescription. It allows you to remain human and support your weight-loss goals.

What to Cheat On

Before we even get to your cheat Rx, let's determine what your food cheats may be. You probably already have an idea of your weaknesses. Below is a list of common cheat foods. Circle any that appeal to you. Note: I am assuming you're going for the full-fat versions of these foods. Some manufacturers have created low-fat or low-sugar versions of their original products, but let's keep this focused on the real things!

Alcohol	Fruit smoothies
Bacon	High-fat meats
Blended coffees (mochaccinos, frappuccinos, ice-blended coffees, and so on)	High-fat salad dressing
Bologna	Hot dogs
Brownies	Ice cream
Butter	Milk shakes
Cakes	Muffins
Candy	Pastries
Chips and crackers	Pies
Chocolate	Pizza
Classic fast-food fare (Big Mac, Whopper, chicken nuggets, and so on)	Processed, packaged sweets (Twinkies, Ding Dongs)
Cookies	Regular cheese

Cream and cream sauces	Regular soda and juice drinks
Cream cheese	Ribs
Croissants	Salami
Dark poultry meat	Scones
Dessert menu items	Sour cream
Doughnuts	Sweet rolls
French fries	Unreasonable amounts of anything*
Fried meats	Whipped cream
Fried vegetables	Whole milk

Unreasonable Amounts of Anything: Can you polish off a whole loaf of bread? Chow down a box of fettuccini or regular pasta with a decadent creamy sauce smothered on top? Eat an entire bag of salty pretzels or organic blue corn chips? It's impossible to list every possible cheat that can run a person's life. Too much of anything can spell trouble, even if it doesn't typically qualify as junk food. So if your particular cheat isn't listed, then use this space to write it down. I'll let you list up to three additional cheats that aren't listed above but that you encounter in your life.

_____

_____

_____

How to Cheat Wisely

My actual cheat prescription is straightforward. You get a total of two cheats per week, and you choose how to allocate them. You may, for instance, need to use two cheats in a single day, leaving you with no more for the rest of the week. Or you may cheat by going to the drive-thru at your favorite fast-food joint one day, and cheat by eating a chocolate bar later that same week. You don't need to limit your cheats to one food or meal. You can mix and match. But try not to exceed two total cheats per week until you've reached your goal weight. Once there, you can add an extra cheat or two into your life. (But again, use common sense; having permission to indulge in three weekly cheats doesn't mean you binge three times a week!)

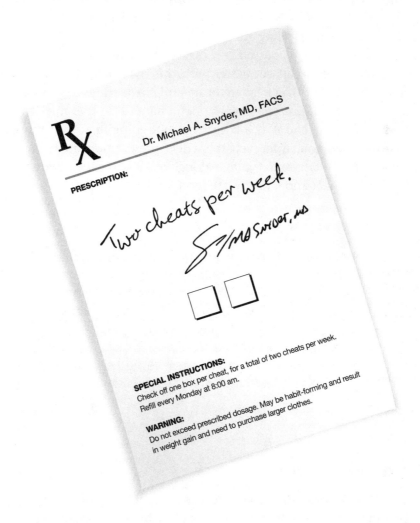

How to Apply

You can apply this cheat prescription to any of your favorite indulgences. Some people feel bad if they don't work out enough. If that's the case, then make a "day off exercise" a cheat. This can be in addition to your food-related cheats. Or, if you're the type who needs to sleep in on Thursday morning rather than go for your regular walk, then check off a box and let go of the guilt. Cheats are all about avoiding feeling guilty!

And don't drive yourself crazy trying to figure out what qualifies as a cheat. You'll get better with this over time. I want you to become your own cheat advocate and cheat referee. Is a table-spoon of peanut butter a cheat? Does a handful of trail mix with white chocolate count as a cheat? I'm not going to answer those questions for you. Approach this cheat prescription broadly for now and then tailor it as you go along. You'll know the difference between a cheat and a legitimate food.

> *A Cheat Trick:* Whenever possible, eat your cheats detached from your real life. By that, I mean don't bring your cheats into your home, work, or car. These places are way too personal and intimate. If you're going to feed the hunger of desire, keep it apart from your everyday life. Stand on the sidewalk of the convenience store and eat them. That will make the foods of temptation seem more like the drugs that they are. The attraction of them will begin to wane.

Unplanned Cheats

We've all been there. A co-worker brings in a box of doughnuts or candy. The houseguest arrives with a huge, decadent dessert from the local bakery that you surely can't avoid. Or you attend a party and though you show up with good intentions to stick with the hearty, wholesome foods on the table, the desserts and delicious deep-fried appetizers are too tempting. What do you do since you've already used up your cheats for the week?

First, take a deep breath. Anytime you encounter a potential unplanned cheat, go ahead and indulge. Satisfy the taste you have for those unexpected cheats, but try to control how much you consume. Take a small serving and walk away. In my doctor's lounge, the world's greatest cookies are always on offer. Each cookie has 400 calories. I can't resist. I grab half of one and then walk away. But I often use cheats as a reward for exercise, and don't feel nearly as bad about taking half a cookie if I've worked out that morning. These are the kinds of choices you, too, will learn to make over time and with practice.

When you do give in to unplanned cheats, especially if you've exceeded your cheats for the week, take some time to think about why they're important to you. Is this a time when you don't want to feel excluded? Do you feel like you're being too restrictive? Are you choosing to eat a favorite food that you find irresistible?

Write down your reasons in your journal. Learn from your experience and move on. One of the most important lessons about cheats is that they don't need to ruin your day. And neither do unplanned cheats as long as you maintain some level of control. Exceeding your cheats doesn't give you permission to eat poorly the rest of the day or week. It's far too easy to "throw away" an entire day or week if you think you've failed your commitment to eating wisely. Let's say, for instance, that you blow the day on Friday because an office party has you eating (and drinking alcohol) to the point you can't even begin to count how many cheats you've used up. Well, if you don't start paying attention again to your eating behavior until Monday, you've basically rewarded yourself with 48 hours of cheating just because of one single misstep. Don't do this to yourself. Think about how this would work in the world of parenting. If you lose your temper on Tuesday and unfairly yell at your daughter over something trivial, would you wait until Monday to be a "good parent" again? Certainly not. We take our jobs and roles as parents seriously, to preserve those important areas in our lives. We should expect the same when it comes to our health and wellness.

Managing Your Screwups

Anyone who is trying to lose weight or start a new exercise program (or, by the same token, establish an intimate relationship, parent a child, or be successful at a project at work) has experienced a screwup. We all define our screwups differently, but they mean the same thing to each of us. It's a time when your best intentions and planning go awry and you act in a way that is contrary to your best-laid plans. Clearly, there are different magnitudes of screwups. Some, like drunk driving, are threatening to your life, health, family, and career. And then there are those screwups with relatively minor significance, such as yelling at your child for something he did when it wasn't really his fault.

Just as I've encouraged you to keep your weight issues in perspective, having a good sense of the magnitude of your screwups and how they affect you is also key. The goal is to limit your screwups consciously and control how they will affect the rest of your life.

Cheats Do Not Equal Screwups

To be absolutely clear: A cheat is not a screwup. A cheat is a planned variance of a "pretty-well-controlled diet and activity regimen." A cheat is expected and planned and a healthy part of the process of controlling weight—it allows you to be human and eliminates the base drive to "do whatever you want to do" all the time by giving you a glimmer of a regular desired indulgence. A screwup, on the other hand, is different; it's often impulsive and always feels wrong. You realize either before, during, or after the screwup that it clearly is a subconscious effort to actively undermine whatever it is you're trying to do to gain control of your life. After a screwup, it's important to define *why* you screwed up, how you can control the damage, how you can take a reality check of its significance, and how you get on with your life in a positive fashion.

It's not uncommon for me to have a patient who is a few years out of surgery gain 20 percent of her excess body weight back. If she loses 140 pounds, for instance, that's a 28-pound weight gain, which is a significant amount of weight with notable impact on self-esteem, health, and life. The first step in counseling this patient is to comfort her and remind her that this is not "an end game." It's not something that has to define her life from this point on. Twenty-eight pounds doesn't mean she will gain the rest of that 140 back. By the time she sees me, though, she has convinced herself that she is back to old habits and is someone who is doomed to be morbidly obese. Remember, the point of surgery is to level the playing field for my patients and give them the same tools that will work for you, the nonmorbidly obese individual.

So when patients begin to gain back weight, I help them get back to basics—to go back to the Rules of the Tool (see Chapter 3). I have them recount for me their recollection of how they should be using their bypass or band procedure. It's amazing that every one of them can do it like they had the surgery yesterday. It's easy for them to remember the rules that they have so readily dismissed from their lives. Often this recounting is a painful process because they realize the simplicity of the process they have abandoned. Then I ask them, "Why haven't you been able to apply these to your life lately?" There is always a good reason: life stresses, financial struggles, habits, familial woes, job difficulties, flare-ups of psychiatric struggles, "just plain laziness," and not wanting to work at it. I then go through with them the same initial step as I did in the beginning:

- Do you remember where you came from?

- Do you have a picture of what you looked like before?

- Do you remember the person you were before you lost the weight?

I make them remember their self-esteem, health challenges, how people treated them, and physical struggles in their life before. I ask: how do you prefer living—as a morbidly obese person or as a normal person? This can be a painful evaluation process. And for all my patients, a life lived with an ability to participate rather than observe is preferable by far. *Doing* is much better than *watching* in life.

Once I get my patients to realize the impact that their recent habits can have on their overall well-being, we then we go through the specific ways in their life that they have brought the maladaptive behavior back, whether it's a renewed routine of going to the coffee shop for a frappuccino, active disregard to volume, bringing poisonous foods back into the house, or letting family and friends who are jealous of their weight loss undermine all their efforts. Many of my patients report a lack of the discipline to plan, which leads to decreased physical activity and an increase in impulse food choices and the volume consumed at meals. All of these percolate into a very real quagmire of screwups. And now the screwup has become a part of their life, which adds a whole other level of disruption to the process.

With these patients I have to slowly and methodically rebuild the simple steps to get them back to who they want to be. The cost of not doing this successfully is not just a size or two, but often a recurrence of diabetes, joint degeneration to the point of needing surgery, sleep apnea and cardiac stress, or once again having to live life with the specter of being seen as someone with "huge weight issues" and all of the social stigmas that implies. You can imagine the desperation of this struggle.

When it comes to managing your own screwups, the first step is not unlike that of my patients': take a reality check to put things into perspective. Ask yourself, what is the real implication of my screwup? Is my eating a whole pound cake really going to change my life? Does it really mean that I'm doomed to failure? Does it mean I should throw out my weight-loss efforts because I've proven to be a slave to pound cake? Am I someone who should never again be trusted and respected because of my carb addiction?

Should my family live in shame because of my inability to avoid the spongy sweets?

You know the answer to all of these questions is a resounding NO!

I know I'm overstating it, and it does seem ridiculous, but it is just that: ridiculous. Gain some perspective. You screwed up. Learn from your mistake and get on with your life. Would you disown a child because he didn't complete a book report on time? Of course not. It's a mistake he should be punished for (maybe) to be more vigilant in the future, but he will still be loved as before. He will still grow up to be a productive, loving, and successful individual. Would you leave your spouse if she backed her car into another car while maneuvering in a parking lot and talking on the cell phone? You'd be angry and it could potentially change your household finances for a bit, but it'll be an event joked about and forgiven in the future. Why are you not as forgiving of yourself for your screwups that revolve around your weight?

Let's go back to the pound cake example: you ate too much pound cake. For mathematical convenience, let's say you ate 14,000 calories (or about ten pound cakes), which equates to four pounds of weight if you do the math: there are 3,500 calories in a pound, so $14,000 \div 3,500 = 4$. Contrary to what you might think, it takes a protracted exposure to excess calories to gain weight, and if that were not the case, then your day of burgers, French fries, and packaged cookies would result in many more pounds gained. Granted, you may feel sick and in a mental fog, but you will not gain four pounds. So get over thinking that you've scorched your earth and "ruined everything." The reality check is that you should stamp the events of that day as a screwup and move on. Forgive yourself as you would anyone else in your life who slips occasionally. A screwup does not mean you're a bad person, or should get depressed over it, or should throw all of your diet and weight aspirations out the window. Once you bring it into this sphere, you can start working on how to start managing and avoiding screwups in the future. And if this is the worst thing that happened to you this year, consider yourself lucky.

My wife can get frustrated with me when I refuse to get emotionally involved or concerned about some of the mishaps that involve our kids, such as our son leaving his homework at school or our daughter not showing enough respect to her grandmother. I have to remind my wife that it's hard for me to get wrapped up in trivial events like that when I have a career requiring me to take someone's life into my hands 20 times a week—to rearrange their anatomy and get them safely back home to their family and friends. It doesn't mean my family isn't important to me, but the reality is the magnitude of risk involved is less, and I'm at a parental advantage because I can keep it in perspective.

So I ask you to do the same. What is hard in your life? What has been hard? Have you lived through the death of good friends, family members, and other loved ones? Have you had relationship difficulties, maybe even divorce? Have you experienced the pain of having family members in the hospital? Have you waited for the results of a scary biopsy or lab report? Have you lost a beloved pet? Have you been on the brink of financial ruin? These are hard things. Very hard. Screwing up by having a dietary dalliance or going a long time without any exercise clearly doesn't register on the radar of life's real struggles and challenges. I need you to keep this in perspective.

Dealing with Foodie ("Toxic") Environments

We all live in a social sphere that requires us to be involved where overindulgence is expected. Think weddings, parties, buffets, and the like. It would be great if we could walk into these environments wearing a hazmat suit so we can view them as toxic as they really are, which would help us avoid accidental exposure to unnecessary foods that have the potential to injure us and veer us off track. A bright orange hazmat suit would also help keep others from coming too close and convincing you to "try this" or "eat that" and basically encouraging you to stuff yourself to the gills with an explosive number of calories. This would make the whole situation a lot easier to deal with, wouldn't it?

In addition to the strategies I briefly covered earlier, following is a list of other ideas that specifically help you to enter these settings with your risks already in check. If you practice any combination of these tools, even if it's just one, you will limit the adverse effects these can have on your good intentions. Remember, don't leave it up to someone else or to chance. Plan your risks as carefully as possible.

Plan Accordingly

Make any invitation to enter a food-filled environment that's hard to control part of your cheat Rx. If you know you're going to Aunt Hilda's house for Thanksgiving, and you're powerless over treats that act like kryptonite to your very being, save all of your week's cheats and then let it go that day. Plan to overindulge and treat it as a cheat—NOT as an impulsive screwup.

Use Fullness to Your Advantage—Beforehand

Ruin your appetite before you go. Christmas cookies don't look half as good at the end of a meal as they did when you first walked in and smelled them. Pre-fill your stomach before entering the toxic environment with a thoughtful, planned meal and hit the door with a level of fullness that gives you control. Do you really care if your cousin Janis is frustrated at you because you didn't eat enough of her meal? I give you permission to tell little white lies if you encounter pushy people who won't let you go from the table empty-handed. Tell these people who lack boundaries that you're not feeling 100 percent, or that you're on antibiotics that prevent you from indulging in certain foods, or you have a food allergy, or that you had a really late lunch. It's okay to lie when it's in your defense. There will be plenty of other people there chomping down and packing it in, and will wake up tomorrow feeling bad. This doesn't have to be you.

Refer back to the full list of foods on pages 95 and 96 to get you the control you need before you even walk in the door. I will

145

regularly have a big glass of water and a filling bar before heading out to a holiday dinner. I don't like the feeling and the hangover I get from the overindulging and the foods that are toxic to my system. People get used to the fact that I'm not an overindulging guy. If they want someone to go hog wild at their party, then they probably shouldn't be inviting me. As I understand it, other than my not being invited because of my personality, this has not been a problem.

Limit Serving Size

Suppose there's a 40-inch lasagna for eight people at a party. There's no law in polite society that says that you have to eat one-eighth of the lasagna. That would be disgusting. Take a small serving using my strategies of volume control and tell the host you'll come back for more later. Then eat your serving and don't go back. You're in charge of how much you put on your plate. Watch out for plate size: party hosts can serve food on big plates. Use small saucers instead if they are available to you.

What happens if you encounter a particularly complicated situation? Let's say you're blessed with an overbearing family member who insists on serving you as if you've just been released from a maximum-security penitentiary and have not had a real meal in 20 years. At this one dinner, she is convinced that you need to make up for the years of denial and calorie restriction that have plagued you. She single-handedly works to undermine any dietary effort you have had over last two decades by giving you an obscene amount of calorie-laden foods. This is where I want you to remember that you're no longer six years old and don't have to clean your plate for fear of punishment. Do some visual and mental gymnastics to actively study your plate, and figure out how much of its contents you want to eat. Feel free to rearrange the plate to allow for a more reasonable intake of the food that has been given to you. Then the two strategies I use are:

1. Try to eat a sensible portion without getting too distracted by conversation, so you stay attuned to how much you're eating. It's often easier to mindlessly plow food

into your mouth if you're multitasking than if you are sitting alone focused solely on eating.

2. Actively avoid sitting and facing the cesspool of temptations for the rest of the meal. Mess up your plate to make it look unappetizing (with the added advantage that it will look like you ate more of it than you really did). And make the food unpalatable. Go ahead and dump salt on your plate to slug-killing levels. Yes, it's wasteful, but it might just save you from yourself.

You would not drive into a rough neighborhood without a plan for how to keep yourself safe. You'd choose the right time of day to make the trip, map out the right path in and out, and keep yourself insulated in a manner that makes you feel safe. This is how you should approach potentially dangerous food neighborhoods.

Plateaus and Weight Gain

I don't know anyone who attempts weight loss and who doesn't hit a wall at some point whereby the weight loss comes to a screeching halt or may even go in reverse. Hitting a plateau is a normal part of the weight-loss process. Let me repeat: a slow-down in your weight loss is to be *expected* as a natural side effect of the process. It's a sign that your body has become more efficient, thus needing less energy (that is, fewer calories) to get more done. The other good news is that it also could be a sign of an invisible transition taking place inside your body: you're still losing fat but you might be retaining water and/or gaining muscle mass.

Also, during this phase your body is learning to operate with less—it's adapting. Giving up any ground at this time can work to make you abandon the good changes you're making. Your body is just now learning that your new control and better dietary and activity changes are not a fluke. As it has been described to me, it's a time when your body is trying to frustrate you by not delivering the results you want. And it's trying to get you back to your

147

overindulgent and more sedentary ways. Do not let the body win this struggle. By persevering and ignoring the scale—and moving ahead as you have planned, the plateau will break and your results will be even more consistent and you will have more control. This is when patience is the doctor's order.

There are other things to consider, though, when the scale starts giving you a hard time. First and foremost, you need to bring your frustrations with your weight loss into the same picture as your expectations. Once you hit a plateau, it's important to ask yourself:

- What are your weight-loss expectations now? Have they changed since you began the weight-loss journey? How have they changed? What's different now?

- Is this plateau really occurring when you're within your goal-weight range? Could you be at a reasonable goal for now and your body is just reminding you of this?

- Are you fighting against an unrealistic expectation of weight loss or an unhealthy goal of "constantly losing weight"?

- Is a plateau part of your endless drive to be caught in a weight-loss struggle?

Again, this goes back to my discussion about you needing to find—and be happy with—an end point to your weight loss. Don't beat yourself up over those last ten pounds. There has to be an end point and it has to be fair-minded for you. I've had patients who reach a size 6 (which they never could have imagined when they first came to me for help in losing the weight), yet they feel the need to be a size 4 once they are at a svelte size 6. Sorry, but for them, being "stuck at a size 6" is not hitting a plateau; and wishing to be a size 4 is plain bad thinking.

If you find yourself hoping, wishing, and dreaming to be just a few pounds lighter than where you are, when your weight is actually quite appropriate, then your wrestle may not be with the weight loss—it's with understanding who you are without a weight-loss struggle.

This is when going back to the exercises I gave you in Part I is key. And if you can't figure out on your own who you are and who you want to be apart from the weight battle, then I recommend reaching out to others and contemplating professional guidance if necessary. A trusted friend, dietitian, or medical professional can give you some perspective in this regard, as well as help you to realize where your weight should be in terms of health and your expectations. Don't get me wrong: I'm not saying that you have a psychiatric illness that needs a diagnosis and treatment, but you may have unrealistic expectations of what your weight-loss goals should be. As I've said, it's not all about the weight loss; it's about getting to the point of using these simple tools to not focus on the weight. It's about getting on with your life. And for many, this experience may be very disruptive to how you define yourself up till now. For those who've lived by the weight of their weight— literally—most of their lives, taking the weight out of the equation can create a huge gap or open space in one's life that now needs to be filled with something else. It can be scary.

Bear in mind that there are realities in weight loss. It always comes in fits and starts. Most weight-loss regimens get going with at least an element of diuresis or water loss. This is what you see with the high-protein diets. You pee up a storm, drop seven pounds in two weeks, and then stall out. That's not a true weight loss. That's a water loss and it's to be expected. A healthy weight loss, on the other hand, involves a slow and steady drop in weight that signifies actual pounds of fat burned. Please don't confuse this with a plateau.

Physiologically, as you lose weight, there will be periods of time when you're changing your body's composition. Your weight can stay the same while you're increasing muscle and decreasing fat. Your clothes will likely fit differently (for the better) but the scale may read the same. Remember that muscle weighs more than fat. During these changes, you need to gauge how you feel.

Often, you will just "feel better" and have more energy. This is to be expected as your diet and behaviors are getting in line with who you want to be and how you want to live your life. Your body will perform better, too.

In my patients, especially ones who have increased their physical activity, I don't worry about a plateau of weight loss until it has persisted for more than six weeks. I'd like to hold you to that same standard. And, as with them, at six weeks of weight stagnation I remind them that this does not mean that you're failing at your weight-loss efforts. It may simply mean that your body is relearning how to metabolize the foods you're feeding it.

I'll also warn you again, however, that this is a dangerous time for you to screw up regularly. As your body goes through this transitional period, it is looking for any excuse to regain the weight it has lost. Overindulging at this time when you're maximally frustrated may result in an explosive weight gain if your body is relieved of the stress of having to figure out how to appropriately use the more limited resources you're giving it. It's like revving an engine before you drive. Your body is warming up for real progress. We have all experienced this when we have gone on a diet program, lost 12 pounds, plateaued, gotten frustrated, reverted back to our old habits, and then gained 20 pounds. That's a predicted routine of giving in to the frustration of a plateau.

If you wait out the six weeks, you've required your body to be more efficient and to effectively use a sparser energy load. When you stoically wait this period out—staying true to your tools despite your disappointment—your discipline will pay off. You will essentially force a reorganizing and rewiring of your physiology that permits your body to give up the fat and maintain a healthier and more efficient lean body mass. Countless times I've fostered my plateau patients through this six-week interval only to receive a cascade of hugs and smiles after the six weeks because the weight loss resumed. Once the corner is turned, there's another drop in weight and clothing size.

When Plateaus Go Beyond Six Weeks

If you don't see the scale tick downward or your clothes fitting better after six weeks of bearing out a plateau, then it's time to take more decisive action. This is especially true if you've noticed a weight *gain* of several pounds in recent weeks. It's possible that the economics of weight loss are not working out for you. Why? Well, as much as I hate to restate old tried-and-true yet overstated dietary and exercise rules, in this scenario you're probably taking in too much and taking out too little. And this could be happening without you even realizing it. In other words, it may be time to reflect more seriously on your physical activity level and dietary habits. Have you been keeping track of your meals and activity levels in your journal? Can you identify times when you've veered farther off track from your tools than you intended?

You need to recalibrate what you're eating, your meal frequency, and volume. Also check your hydration and your activity level. Are you drinking more calories in the form of sugary sodas, alcohol, or juice drinks? How ambitious is your activity level? Do you sweat? Do you engage in some form of physical activity at least three days a week? Or are you living a sedentary life but allowing yourself to have a full fare of cheats per week? The answers to these questions can make for sobering news.

But the good news is if you're on a plateau for an extended period of time, anything will help. Being at a stable weight for a protracted period of time is a gift of sorts. You have cleanly and clearly defined the very efficient machine that you are and you're in perfect balance. A stable or unchanging weight means that you have ideally balanced your intake and output. I say that this is a gift because you have expertly proven that anything you do now will result in a weight/calorie deficit. If you do anything to nudge along your weight loss, it will pay off directly. Just eliminating 200 calories of soda per day will directly translate into a 21-pound weight loss in a year! That is phenomenal and very "real" math. All by just eliminating a soda. I've broken plateaus like this for my patients just by dropping their carbohydrate intake from 40 percent to 30 percent of their overall diet and increased their activity level by ten minutes a day. It doesn't take much—it just takes *something*.

In principle, if you can tweak one thing about your diet and one thing about your physical activity routine, you can have an impact and break through. Your body is dying for the opportunity to be more efficient. By improving how you live your life up to and through the plateau period, you've already made great strides in increasing the efficiency of your body's machinery. Now you just have to up the ante and put a higher-quality fuel into it. Pushing past a plateau and continuing to see results may entail increasing the intensity of your workouts (much more on workouts coming up in the next chapter) and pushing your body just a little bit harder. Keeping the body guessing is what keeps you moving forward and not letting it get used to your workouts. On the dietary front, check in with your choices and make sure you haven't been sidelining the tools and going back to old habits.

Plateau-Breaking Tools: The essence of breaking through a long plateau boils down to reminding yourself of the main tenets of the tools. Chances are, you've let one or more of these tools fall off the radar. When you hit a stubborn plateau, see if you can change just one thing about your diet, and one thing about your physical activity. The following guidelines will help you:

- *Remove a cheat from your weekly allowance.* Or, check to see if you've been letting your cheats bloom to more than two per week. If so, just cut back your cheat to a sensible two times per week and make sure you're recording them as you use them. The enemy of weight loss is the food you eat spontaneously. It is almost always eaten without hunger. It is an impulse item. So, if you need to cheat, then plan the what, when, and why of eating the particular food.

- *Substitute your caloric beverages with plain unflavored water (regular or sparkling).* If you choose to have a "diet" drink that has zero calories, aim to drink beverages that don't contain aspartame, which has been shown in some studies to trigger hunger and cravings for real sugar and disrupt your brain's full headquarters to know when enough is enough. Make it a goal to have 60 to 80 ounces (2 to 2.5 quarts, or 1.75 to 2.5 liters) of water per day.

- *Be sure you're eating five to six meals per day.* Eating about every three hours is just right—feel free to eat at 7 and 10 A.M., then again at 1, 4, 7, and 10 P.M. Set your watch to remind you. Carry your meals with you. Plan. If you are not eating your meals frequently, your body thinks that you're depriving it and it holds on to the fat. If you give your body frequent, small, high-quality protein meals, you "trick" it into giving up fat.

- *Don't eat blindly until you feel full.* Have you stopped visually measuring out your meals on a plate and gotten cavalier about volume control? Remember, your brain is on a 20-minute delay from your stomach. So, if you eat until you "feel full," you're more likely to eat 20 minutes too long. So, measure the appropriate amount of food on a plate, eat it, sit back for 20 minutes, and you will feel full. Make sure to stay mindful in the eating process by avoiding distracting settings such as those that include a television, computer, or even talking on the phone. This bears repeating: this isn't a good time for multitasking.

- *Watch what you eat; clock it out.* Aim for your meals to be built around high-quality, dense protein and fibrous vegetables and fruits. I like to use the clock analogy as a way to portion out your meals on the plate. Vegetables should take up the space from 12 o'clock to 6 o'clock. Lean protein should take up the space from 6 o'clock to about 10. The remaining time between 10 and 12:00 is reserved for the grains and starches. Limit the amount of processed "white" foods—rice, bread, pasta, potatoes, and baked goods—in your allowance of starches and grains.

- *Beware of unhealthy and excessive protein shakes and bars.*
  Have too many of these snuck into your life? There is
  a big misunderstanding in the market today regard-
  ing protein shakes. People drink them thinking they
  are good for them, but they can be one of the highest
  calorie and sugar sources of anything you will consume.
  This is why I created one of the lowest calorie shakes on
  the market. If you enjoy ready-to-drink shakes, make
  sure you find one that is under 150 calories and contains at least 10 grams of protein. Or follow the recipe
  on page 87. Protein bars are okay as meals, but they are
  not a "free" food to be eaten at your leisure. The best
  ones contain protein that is twice the amount of carbs
  and have minimal saturated and trans fats. I'd rather
  you have a protein shake than miss a meal. However,
  if you've introduced protein shakes (or any shakes for
  that matter) into your life, you need to quickly do the
  math to make sure that they fit with your activity levels
  and dietary goals. Many are formulated for performance
  athletes, are designed to be meal replacements, and may
  have too many calories. Many have multiple servings
  per container—so you are unwittingly taking in multiple meals at each sitting. If you need extra protein, I
  like the drinks that contain only protein with low or no
  carbs. But unless you're really going hard at an aerobic
  or bodybuilding routine, you shouldn't need all that
  extra protein. Try not to stray too far from my shake
  recipes, which are formulated to be low in calories and
  high in nutrition. Ahem: they are not the same as a trip
  to DQ or Jamba Juice!

- *Police your snacking.* How much are you eating in between those five or six meals per day? There is really no
  time for snacking if you're eating meals throughout the
  day. If you need a particular snack food, work it into
  your next meal. For example, if on rare occasion (!) you
  need five Doritos, then eat them as carbs at your next

meal—you know, in that space between 9 o'clock and 12 o'clock.

- *Stop and think again.* As always, if you have concerns about a food item or a meal issue, do not put your health at risk. Stop and think, is it worth it? If you need additional coaching in the above rules and/or how to adapt them to your life, then please go to my Website, www.fullbar.com.

Once again, I'm trying to redefine how you view your life and keep your weight-loss efforts in perspective. I'm not interested in a minute-by-minute counting of your dietary habits. What I'm interested in is a reconfiguring of how you view yourself and how you gain control. I don't care about minor weight fluctuations through the week. It's critical that you weigh yourself once every two weeks maximum, at the same time of day, same place, wearing the same clothes (or naked), and on the same scale. If you are tempted to weigh in more often than that, have someone hide the scale. If possible, weigh yourself away from your home. My patients can only weigh themselves inside my office.

Be Full and Healthy

How you live your life and approach your issues with weight will no doubt affect every single person you come into contact with. Though you may be reading this book specifically for the purpose of losing weight, I hope that by the end of it you'll have shifted to a much broader perspective that honors the health component over any other in achieving a certain waist size. And learning how to shoulder the weight of disappointments, setbacks, and new challenges will be part of your transformation. I don't know anyone who doesn't live a full life without some hiccups along the way. They are, after all, what make up a full and healthy—human—life.

The Full Challenge: Day 6

Today, make it a goal to plan your cheats for the following two weeks. Take note of your calendar and social obligations when you do this exercise. It helps to know, for instance, that you have a dinner party on Saturday night for which you'll likely need to use one of your cheat prescriptions. Or perhaps you have your son's birthday party on Sunday afternoon that will require some leeway. One thing to keep in mind as you plan: try not to use both of your cheats over the weekend. If you save up your cheats for the weekend, you're more likely to binge or splurge at some other point during the week, as this will start to feel like a traditional restrictive diet.

Reminder: You must plan your cheats 24 hours in advance. The cheat prescription is straightforward. You get two cheats per week, and you choose how to allocate them. You do not need to limit your cheats to one type of food or meal. You can mix and match but they must be planned. For example, if you're dying to have that hamburger from your favorite fast-food joint, you must schedule the visit during the previous day. *No impulse cheating*, like taking a handful of candy from your co-worker's desk.

JANET CARPENTER

Age: 51, Height: 5'9"
Starting: Weight: 198.8, Size: 14
Final: Weight: 181.8, Size: 12
Total Lost: 17 Pounds and 17"

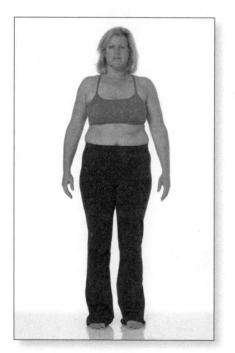 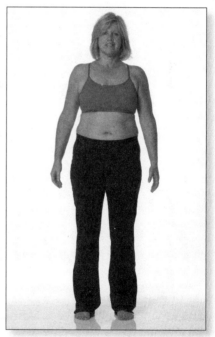

"As an interior designer, my image is important. I carry my weight in the middle, and I realize that at my age, hormones make weight loss more challenging. But I'm losing the weight and finding the plan so easy to follow. I make my own healthy meals at night and use my cheats to have a glass of wine with dinner."

PART III

Be Full,
Live Full

CHAPTER SEVEN
DAY 7

MOVE FORWARD
ONE FULL DAY AT A TIME

Eight months and 130 pounds after bariatric surgery, Mark S. came to see me for a checkup. When I asked him what his secrets were, he said, "I love cookies, but frankly, I have had more than enough cookies in my day. I have eaten enough for multiple people! It's okay for me to take some time off. Heck, and that goes for pasta, too." I loved his realistic assessment of what his weaknesses are and what compromises he is willing to make.

This change won't be easy, but it will be easier than any other diet you've ever tried. Now that you've gained a new perspective and a wealth of strategies, it's time to cover the physical secrets to really making this work.

Fitting in the Physical Ingredients to Weight Loss

Can you lose weight without slugging it out in an exercise routine?

Yes.

And no.

This is perhaps one of the most commonly asked questions I get. While you can control the weight-loss math with diet alone, it's not the best—nor the easiest, healthiest—way to go. The body, after all, is built to move through space. And when you combine eating properly with exercise, the results can be limitless if not magical.

It's common knowledge that exercise is good for you, and may be one of the best things you can do for your overall health. You've heard about the benefits over and over, from how it can lower your risk for a multitude of diseases, including diabetes, cancer, heart disease, depression, and osteoporosis, to how it helps you to sleep better, improve your mood, infuse you with energetic feelings, stave off dementia in old age, and boost immunity. And you also are probably aware that exercise helps you to burn more calories and lose weight more quickly. But you still might not understand *why*.

First, exercise increases your metabolism as you're working out, and metabolism can remain at an elevated state long afterward (called the "afterburn"). This allows you to burn more calories and move fat out of cells for energy. Second, exercise helps you to maintain—and build—lean muscle mass, which is critical to your ability to burn fat. By increasing your lean muscle mass, you'll give yourself an even greater capacity to burn more calories throughout the day and keep your metabolism running high.

The value of muscle mass is often ignored as people worry so much about fat. But when it comes to quality of life, longevity, and the ability to maximize metabolism, it's all about muscle. Unlike fat, muscle is a high-maintenance tissue; it requires a lot of energy to keep it in good working order. This explains why lean, more muscular people have an easier time burning calories at rest than people with higher proportions of body fat. People also don't think about the fact that muscles have functions other than just allowing us to voluntarily move and lift heavy objects. Consider all of the involuntary muscle activities that go on 24/7: your heart, which itself is a muscle, pumps oxygen and nutrients to cells; breathing depends on muscles to deliver oxygen; muscle action pumps white blood cells through your lymphatic system as part of your immune system; and muscle activity in the skin allows us to sweat and maintain our temperature. Needless to say, muscle is in constant use by the body to keep it alive and well—hence, muscle burns calories, whereas fat just stores them. So you can see why the more lean muscle you have, the faster your metabolism will be. It's the main determinant of your metabolism's speed. Is it sprinting at a hundred miles an hour or crawling at a fraction of that rate?

The muscle factor is partly why age and weight are so interconnected. Every year after age 25, most of us gain one pound of body weight, yet lose a third to a half pound of muscle. It's no wonder that our resting metabolism decreases approximately 0.5 percent every year. So unless we downshift our caloric intake as our metabolisms decelerate, we'll experience weight gain. Although losing a fraction of muscle mass each year may seem minuscule, it adds up to be quite significant—about a 1 to 2 percent loss of strength each year. And with this loss of muscle strength, we tend to spontaneously become less active because daily activities become more difficult and exhausting to perform. Sound familiar? It's a fact of life and a prime reason why people have a harder time managing their weight after they've been declared "over the hill." It's not your imagination that it's more challenging to control your weight if you're over 40 or 50, and the battle of the bulge only seems to only get tougher with each passing year. You can have a big impact, though, if you prevent the massive drop-off of muscle mass by adding routine activity to your life.

Third, the muscles you work and build through exercise will set off a sequence of events. They will, for instance, require more oxygen to work efficiently and will command that the body meets certain demands. The muscles' work and recovery will also help your body make and use more growth hormone—which will again make it easier to continue with your muscle development and maintenance. What this ultimately means is you will foster a stronger cardiovascular system high on the metabolism meter.

That said, I'll do my best to avoid the term *exercise* because I know that it makes some people cringe. I have only three goals that need to be met when you ultimately become versed in doing physical activity: if done properly, physical activity requires a change of clothes into workout gear, sweating to the point of needing a shower, and being unable to talk in full sentences while doing it.

This can seem very scary for people who have led sedentary lives, who don't like to sweat, who fear failing at a routine exercise program, who fear their body's response (that is, elevated heart rate, hard breathing, muscle soreness), who think they don't have access to proper exercise, who don't think they can afford it, who don't know what to do, who are too tired and busy, who fear they are going to die, who fear it will hurt, or who merely don't want to look stupid and be embarrassed.

Plan, Ritual, Religion

I once had a patient who refused to exercise. She hit a plateau 40 pounds above where she wanted to be after losing more than 100 pounds after band surgery. Without physical activity, she couldn't get closer to her goal. So we started to talk about her predicament and figure out what she could do to reverse this trend. I found out she lived less than a mile from her local gym and it would cost $55 to join for one month, which was something she could afford. I gave her the following two-week assignment: buy a one-month membership and on her way home from work, Monday through Friday, she was to stop at this gym, slap her hand on the check-in counter in the entranceway, go back to her car, and drive home. She was not allowed to go through the entrance gate.

After two weeks of following my instructions, she came back and said, "I don't think that was very much exercise." I said, "You did the hardest part of working out: getting to gym five days a week!" She had used every excuse in book prior to this assignment, but I knew that 90 percent of the difficulty is *getting* to the gym. She proved she could get there. Check.

Over the next two weeks, I added another assignment: I had her step onto one of the treadmills and go as slow as she wanted, for three full minutes at a time wearing street clothes and her regular work shoes. Two weeks later, she reported back that she found the three minutes boring and could go farther. I said, "Now you've done the second hardest thing: getting on a piece of equipment at the gym." For the next two weeks, I had her walk eight minutes and change into sneakers before doing so, but allowed her to still wear her street clothes. She came back again two weeks later and again said that she wanted to increase her workout time. I congratulated her, telling her that she'd worked out more than most people I knew in the last six weeks!

Next, I encouraged her to change into gym clothes and I built her workouts up 2 minutes a day until she was able to go three miles without stopping on the treadmill at a 15-minute-per-mile pace. She started with 8-minute sessions and it took her 19 weeks to get to three miles, by increasing her exercise time by 2 minutes per week.

If you're like most people reading this, you're probably thinking that this was a colossal waste of time because it's such a slow process. How did this woman tolerate it? Well, for this patient it was the farthest she'd gone in her life. We created a plan (phase 1) that established a ritual (phase 2) that then allowed her to accept this new routine as a part of her life, like a religion (phase 3). At the beginning of this experience, "exercise" was the furthest thing from her mind. She had never enjoyed working out, and being at the gym with sweaty people and wearing stinky clothes was not on her radar. And now she is one of them.

Taking a full 19 weeks to get to a regular three-mile workout may seem so slow as to be fruitless. But wait: isn't that the negative brain talking? Her success happened a lot faster than if she had not ever started. And, the time spent building her level of performance was not wasted. She rebuilt her behaviors, interest, motivation, execution, and fitness all quite gently and elegantly. In fact, I'd say her transformation was more impressive than that of a daily jogger into a marathoner. She started from nothing and was a deeply committed *non*-exerciser. To start from there and move to a life of activity and regular healthful pursuits is nothing short of heroic.

So I ask you: can you walk into a gym and slap your hand on the counter? If you can, you're ready to start a workout routine.

And if you don't want to join a gym, can you drive to the mall? How many laps around the mall can you do? Can you walk up one flight of stairs? Can you park two spots away from where you usually do? Can you take your dog (who is dying for more attention) two houses farther on your evening walk?

I've got a program for everyone, whether you're the one with a litany of legitimate excuses or a seasoned active person with a regular routine. Being active is part of leading a Full life. My three-phase program outlined below will bring out the inner athlete in you, showing you how to find the easiest, cheapest, least fearful, and most convenient activity imaginable. As much as this book is a departure from a traditional diet, so too is this section on exercise. What you will find, just as you have been finding all along, is the guidance to find the creative solutions that work for you as an individual.

Phase 1: Planning

In my experience, most people don't come home from work and sit on the couch, just for fun, contemplating exercise. And how many people do you know who jump up at the spur of the moment and go work out? Probably not many. It's critical that you plan your activity. We're like all other forces of nature. A body at rest tends to stay at rest, and when we do move, we like to take the path of least resistance.

If you do not plan your activity changes and increases, they will never occur. When you drive to the mall, for instance, you have to actively think about where you're going to park because you'll naturally drive to the spot closest to the entrance. You have to actively plan to walk up the stairs to your second-floor office, or you'll simply use the elevator. The planning is critical. I always tell people who want to actively engage in more vigorous activity that the best way to do it is to set up everything in your favor so you don't have to exert much thought about getting it done.

Let me give you a personal example. As I detailed earlier, during my residency I didn't work out at all and gained weight. When

I tried to bring activity back into my life by going to the gym after work, I showed up about once a week at the start. But what I really liked was the coffee bar at the gym, though it was not helping my waistline. The length of my days were often unpredictable, and long. I had a young family at home waiting to see me and if I didn't see them in the evenings, I wouldn't see them at all. I had no interest in doing more physically, so I had to make a change. My ritual became as follows:

I pack a gym bag with my work clothes for the day in my car the night before. I lay my workout clothes near my bed in their anatomic position before I go to sleep. I set three alarms and stagger their times to make sure I get up. Upon awakening, I use the bathroom, brush my teeth, dress into my gym clothes, and get into my car. Not once do I even hesitate to ponder if I want to work out or not, because the answer would be *no*. My rule is I can put off going to the gym only after I drive out of my driveway. And by then, I'm thinking that I'm too awake so I can't turn back. I've taken myself out of the equation entirely. I never think of whether or not I want to go to the gym. It's nonnegotiable at that point. I've grown to love working out, and today it's part of my DNA.

Most of us can be highly motivated to work out the night before we plan to do so, but then by morning we no longer feel that same motivation. That's why it's critical to do all the planning in that highly motivated state and then plan to also get past those moments when you know you'll want to stay in bed and ditch the workout entirely. My morning brain has no desire to do anything but stay in my warm bed and sleep longer.

Find a way to bring activity into your life that will become a routine and then eventually a religion, or that can create a baseline for you to then explore other ways of engaging in physical activity. Ritual first, then religion. For some, just walking to your mailbox and back every day and incrementally adding blocks to your walk over time can result in a serious workout. One patient of mine added just 50 yards a day to her walks; at the end of three months she was walking close to three miles. She rewarded herself with her first pair of walking shoes and a year later, was training for her first marathon. When she told me she felt like an athlete, I reminded her that she was an athlete to me the first day she walked 50 yards.

Here are some ideas to consider if you're currently sedentary and need a plan to just get going:

- Walk to your mailbox and back to your front door five times.

- Walk around your block two times. Add five to ten minutes more on a daily or weekly basis.

- March in place during commercials when watching television.

- Go to a group exercise class with a friend as a guest.

- Go to your local park and walk its paths.

- Every time you park with the intent to shop, park as far away from the destination as possible.

- If you work on the 15th floor, get off on the 14th floor and walk the stairs.

None of these activities will kill you, embarrass you, or break the bank. But they all will teach you a valuable lesson: you can change your behavior for physical good without taking drastic measures. Because it's been proven to take about 21 days to create—and, conversely, break—a habit, make it a goal to engage in physical activity for 21 straight days. By the 22nd day, you'll need it. Then, hopefully, and despite your present skepticism, you will become one of those "annoying" people who loves to do activity and "feels off" if you don't get your activity fix. The body is a remarkable machine: if a completely sedentary person walks around the block at a good clip, he'd be much fitter the next day because his cells will have responded in ways that are seemingly unimaginable. Don't underestimate the power of the human body in movement.

So, where do you go from here? The options are limitless. Once you've accomplished just one full activity, such as walking around your block twice, see if you can double that task by adding another lap or two. Eventually, there will come a time when you realize that you're doing real work and your body is doing better as well. It becomes more comfortable with the activity. I know that you're thinking: *I'll be 80 years old at this rate before I'm truly "exercising" like I probably should be.* The problem is not the rate at which you increase your activity. It's that you haven't started yet!

Here's another way to look at it: one mile equals 5,280 feet. If you walk 59 feet per day, which is probably closer than the distance to your mailbox, and if you add 59 feet a day, in 90 days you'll be walking a mile. In one year you'll be walking four miles. Again, this may seem slow to you in terms of how far you're progressing, but what's your rush? I'm not interested in how unimpressive it is that you walked 59 feet on January 1. I'm more impressed that you walked a mile on March 31. You probably won't break a sweat until sometime deep in February, but by the end of March you may want to buy some fancy shoes.

Commit to find out what exercise you want to do physically and try to do it five days per week. Do not be afraid of joining a real class (for example, step, yoga, spinning, whatever). Every evening you plan the what and when and where of the next day's activity. Remember, plan first, then do what you plan.

Once you're in a routine of working out five days a week, plan your off days. These don't always have to be on the weekend. It can be hard to get back into your workout routine on a Monday morning if you haven't exercised since Friday. Scatter your off days and use your personal calendar to schedule your "relax" days around your responsibilities. Some days are crazier than others so be prepared for them.

Phase 2: Making It a Ritual

You're an athlete when you get up the next day to do something physical again or when you can't catch your breath for a few minutes, which may scare you a little. Your body was designed to increase its conditioning and tolerance to stress of a physical nature. Even NFL players and Olympic athletes go to training camps after hiatuses from their routines to get back into shape. These athletes are patient with their training and don't try to overdo it on the first day, or during the first week for that matter. It's perfectly fine to go slow.

Once you get into a routine, you'll join the ranks of those who exercise regularly. These are the folks who maintain a ritual that has them engaged in physical activity most days of the week, though they may not be going as hard as they can to test their limits. If you've established a comfortable ritual, you may need to increase the intensity of your workouts to keep your body guessing and burning maximally. Some ideas:

- Add more total minutes to your workouts.

- Add more resistance and/or intensity. For example, if you're enjoying a machine at the gym (elliptical, stationary bike, and so on) increase its resistance or incline and go for longer periods. Even one minute of increased intensity makes a huge difference. If your workouts are spent walking outdoors, walk faster and find challenging paths uphill and downhill. Carry three- or five-pound weights in your hands.

- Try something totally new to your body. Shock it! Step onto a machine you've never tried at the gym, go to a class you've never explored before, or take a dancing class. Dancing can burn 975 calories per hour! It's okay to feel sore for a few days afterward (see below).

- Add a weight-training portion to your cardio routine. You can start with the puny weights. They still count and are more than you are doing now, right? They are a great start.

The Full Strength: Fitness buffs love to talk about strength training for good reason: it helps increase muscle mass, strength, and bone health. These benefits are not as strongly associated with aerobic exercise, which improves cardiovascular fitness and burns calories. In fact, strength training can provide up to a 15 percent increase in your metabolism; the bonus is that it also aids the body's use of fat for hours after exercise. This "afterburn" keeps going for longer than you're working out. Strength training is not only an effective antidepressant and sleep enhancer, it has also been shown to increase bone mass, which is extremely important for maintaining bone density later in life and reducing your risk for fractures and osteoporosis. The muscles you engage when you put pressure on your bones forces them to get stronger. In fact, recent studies have shown that loss of bone density may be a better predictor of death from atherosclerosis (hardening of the arteries) than cholesterol levels.

The thought of strength training needn't be intimidating. It can be done with an inexpensive set of free weights (for example, barbells and dumbbells) or with equipment found at your local gym that works various parts of your body in a more controlled way.

Aim to work your muscles this way two or three times a week for about 30 minutes each time, and avoid using weights every day—an every-other-day schedule allows your muscles to recover. Try not to exercise the same muscles two days in a row. Because improvement in any muscle tone and function results from stressing and recovering the muscle, it also pays to challenge yourself and feel sore once in a while. When you work out hard enough to make your muscles burn, that sensation is a sign that you are stressing your muscles. Within the next day or two, your muscles will feel sore and achy to the touch or with movement because they are recovering. Scientists call this DOMS, or delayed onset muscle soreness.

We used to think that next-day muscle soreness was caused by a buildup of lactic acid in muscles, but now we know that it's caused by damage—microscopic tears—to the muscle fibers themselves, which is actually a good thing in this case. It turns

171

out that this muscle pain is a normal response to unusual exertion and is part of an adaptation process that leads to greater stamina and strength as the muscles recover and build bigger cells. It's not the same as the muscle pain or fatigue you experience during exercise. This delayed pain is also very different from the acute, sudden pain of an injury such as a muscle strain or sprain, which is marked by an abrupt, specific, and sudden pain during activity and often causes swelling or bruising. So yes, there's something to be said for the adage "No pain, no gain."

Finding the balance between pushing yourself hard and risking injury is key to any workout. Remember that you don't have to train like an Olympic athlete to gain fitness. Use next-day muscle soreness as a rough guide to getting and staying in shape. Go out one day and work hard enough to feel the burn, and then back off. You can create intervals of intensity for yourself based on your perceived rate of exertion. This can entail simply power walking on hills. Climb a hill at a good clip until your muscles feel stiff, and then slow down your pace or turn around and cruise downhill. Depending on how sore your muscles feel, take the next day off, try another exercise that engages a different set of muscles, or go at a very slow pace. Do not attempt to get that burning sensation back during exercise until the soreness has gone away completely.

Most competitive athletes work out very hard only once or twice a week. The best weight lifters lift very heavy weights only once every two weeks per body part. High jumpers jump for height only once a week. Shot-putters throw for distance only once a week. Remember: The recovery process is just as important as the workout itself. In many ways, it's part of the workout itself, so don't forget about it.

Conquer Your Fears

Millions of us resolve to "get more active," but then we keep up our new routine for just a few weeks. You don't remember when you fell off the wagon, but it happened. And now you may be fearing that failure again—hoping I've got a secret formula for making this exercise thing finally work this time.

Giving you a specific (100 percent guaranteed!) exercise protocol is beyond the scope of this book. By this point, if you're looking for me to give you an exercise program, you're missing the message. My hope for you is that you align what you love to do with being more physically active. Just like I won't tell you exactly what to eat and not eat, I won't force you to participate in exercise x, y, or z. The secret is to be active for pleasure.

See if you can be motivated less by exercise's body-sculpting rewards and more by how it makes you feel. That's all you really need to stay in the game.

Choose one activity this week and plan to do more of that activity. Remember, it doesn't have to be a Herculean effort or come under the traditional category like joining a gym or suddenly becoming the neighborhood jogger. Give yourself permission to move away from traditional formats of exercise that have never worked for you in the long run, and open yourself up to exploring opportunities to get active in other, more creative ways that really move you from the inside out. You'll keep coming back to doing them repeatedly.

Go easy at the start and just get your circulation moving faster and for longer and longer periods of time. Schedule daily walks or call a friend in the morning and ask, "What can we do today?" Do jumping jacks and stretch in front of the television rather than lying on the couch. Plan a Saturday night dancing with your spouse or a group of friends. If you don't belong to a gym, ask a co-worker who is a member to take you to his or her favorite group exercise class. You never know, you just might fall in love with it. For many people, the problem is not so much the start part as it is the sustaining part.

I've heard every excuse and so have you. I've used them a lot myself! I think the top two excuses are the commitment (time, energy, convenience, and so on) and the body's response (sweating, increased heart rate, joint pain, shortness of breath, dizziness, achy muscles). Let's see if the following thoughts don't help out in this complaint department.

I don't have time to exercise: Does anybody really have time for exercise? As with anything else in life, you won't have time for exercise unless you plan for it. Just ten minutes here and ten minutes there, or changing how you park a car in a lot, can make a difference. I don't know anyone who can't find ten extra minutes a day if not several pockets of time throughout the day and opportunities to put some muscle into the daily grind (walking faster, taking stairs two at a time, and so on). It's perfectly fine to go slow and steady when you come out of the gates in establishing a routine. Once you understand (and physically feel) the value that exercise can bring to your life, you will find a way to carve out time no matter how busy your schedule gets. And don't fall into the trap of thinking that your workout program has to be completed every day in one continuous segment.

All the research indicates that you get the same health benefits by doing, say, three 10-minute bouts of exercise as you would from doing a single 30-minute workout. So if you're short on time some days, go right ahead and break up your routine in manageable pieces. If you're going to succeed on your workout program, you'll have to adapt to the changes in your schedule, so be creative in finding ways to make exercise a part of your life. And always do something you enjoy or at least do not hate.

I'm too tired to exercise: Experiment with exercising at different times of the day, and try shifting the bulk of your workouts to the early morning hours, when the day's obligations and distractions haven't begun to either disrupt you or wear you down. Make sure you're getting enough sleep, too. The first five minutes can be the hardest, but once you get over that initial hump, the body takes over. And if you do find yourself chronically tired, then I'd stop to ask why. Chronic exhaustion isn't a sign of good health. You would do well to examine your lifestyle, priorities, and attempts to reduce your stress load. Although there are bound to be legitimate excuses to avoid physical activity, many of them fall under the psychological category. In other words, they are associated with your fears and feelings of inadequacy or embarrassment.

I don't like exercise; I find it boring: Given the number of options for getting more active today, I don't understand this excuse. Why would you force yourself to engage in any activities that bore you or mentally drain you? Gyms and group exercise classes are not for everyone. Engaging in the same routine every time you work out also isn't for everyone. Ruts ("same time, same place") can get tedious and uninspiring. Getting physical should be invigorating. As soon as you get your circulation going, those feelings of "I'm bored and tired" usually fade away as endorphins begin to take over. Stop thinking of it as drudgery and view it as time for yourself. We all lead stressful, busy lives. Making more time for yourself should be a bonus!

When I trained for a marathon, I invented the *"Sopranos* workout" so I could advance from being a casual runner barely able to grind out two miles to someone who could endure the long haul. I always wanted to watch this popular television series, but it was in the final season by the time I got the bug to watch it. And I also wanted to run a marathon when I turned 40 years old. So I bought the whole series, and my rule was that I could only watch it if I was actually running on the treadmill, which for me wasn't an inherently interesting activity. Even when I didn't want to run, I really wanted to see what Tony and company were up to. So, I plowed through six full seasons, and by the time I reached the end I could run for two full shows—100 minutes. Then, I moved on to my next series. Right now I'm watching *Weeds* after just finishing *Nip/Tuck* and *Entourage*. I don't love to run. But it's a way that I can legitimize watching TV I never have time for—and get a workout in.

I didn't get the results I wanted, so I gave up: When someone brings this up, I question how committed they were to finding what they love to do that gets them more active, sticking with a regular regimen, and giving it time for the body to respond. Remember, from the moment you start making shifts in how you eat and "activate," your body will be undergoing a multitude of invisible changes at the cellular level, all of which build up and set a strong foundation for dramatic future results. Remember that we're not aiming for just weight loss. We're seeking so much more. Robust cardiovascular and immune systems. More lean muscle mass. Rejuvenating sleep. A lower risk for weight-related health conditions such as type 2 diabetes and high blood pressure. A strong skeletal system that supports other systems and organs. A lower risk for age-related diseases and a slowdown in the degenerative process that affects everything.

I don't like how exercise makes me feel—short on breath, sweaty, and sore: The effects of physical exertion are different for everyone depending on their conditioning, and it's a universal experience to go through a "breaking-in" period whereby you're not feeling 100 percent. This is especially true when you start a program or intensify an existing routine by taking it to the next level. This is a normal part of the process, and though your body's response may make you uncomfortable, it shouldn't frighten you. I'm not asking you to get so out of breath that you're on the verge of fainting or throwing up. Use your instincts to know when to push harder and when to back off.

Sweating is your body's way of keeping your temperature normal as you exert energy; it's also a sign that you're doing something good for yourself! If sweating bothers you enough to avoid any activity that has you dripping, then opt for water sports like swimming or aqua aerobics. And as for feeling sore following a session of exercise, again this is your body's way of recovering so you can go harder and longer the next time. It's a positive sign—not a negative. On days that particular muscles feel heavy and achy, don't use them and focus on other muscle groups. Give your muscles a few days to recover after you've worked them well. Remember, muscle pain after a workout is a normal response to unusual exertion and is part of an adaptation process that leads to greater stamina and strength as the muscles recover and build more powerful tissues.

Once you get used to the effects of exercise, they won't seem so terrible. The more fit you become, the easier your exercises will feel and the more you'll want to further challenge your body. Remember, too, that as your fitness level increases, your capacity to work your body harder and burn more calories will increase naturally as you gain fat-burning muscle mass. Take it slow and steady. Soon enough, the benefits will start to outweigh the cons that you initially have toward exercise and you'll begin—believe it or not—to look forward to sweating, breathing hard, and feeling sore!

Phase 3: Practice Your Religion

In this phase, you've succeeded in establishing a regular routine and are enjoying the fruits of your labor. You've also gotten good about knowing when to push yourself a little harder and when to back off. You may even contemplate the following:

- Sign up for a local charity event, such as a 5K or 10K walk/run.

- Train for a sprint-distance triathlon.

- Start a running, cycling, or hiking group in your community.

- Sign up for a half marathon or even a full marathon.

- Become a certified instructor for a class and start teaching and motivating others at your local gym.

You'll be amazed at what you can do when you have a consistent routine and are fully tuned in to your body's physical capacity and limitations. Here are some final tips and reminders to consider in bringing out your inner athlete:

- *Be reasonable.* Don't commit to working out every day. You won't do it. Commit to three days per week to start. And limit your exertion to what is within reason for you. You know your limits. Just 20 minutes here, a stair climb there, and 10 minutes lifting weights in front of the television a few times a week can have immediate impacts.

- *Expand your workout reasonably, too.* Add effectiveness to your workout by increasing variety or intensity or time. You don't have to go full-out every day of the week for an obscene number of hours.

- *Have fun.* If you hate something, you won't do it. Find out what you like or seek it out. Try new things merely because they sound like they'd be fun. Experiment. There are thousands of activity options—if you never find one for you and try them all, then you are already a pretty darn active person. Don't force yourself to engage in any activities that bore you or mentally drain you. Gyms and group exercise classes are not for everyone. Also bear in mind that exercise is invigorating. As soon as you get your circulation going, those feelings of "I'm too tired" usually fade away as endorphins begin to take over. Try moving your workouts to the morning, when the day's events haven't kicked in to disrupt you or wear you down. The first five minutes are the hardest, but once you get over that initial hump, the body takes over. And if you do find yourself chronically tired, then I'd stop to ask why. Chronic exhaustion isn't a sign of health. You would do well to examine your lifestyle, priorities, and attempts to reduce your stress load.

- *Commit.* Reward yourself for meeting your goals, such as by treating yourself to an afternoon or just an hour spent engaging in whatever activity or hobby brings you pleasure. Don't punish yourself if your attempts at exercise don't get done exactly as planned. As with weight-loss goals, one day missed does not mean you should throw out the whole week. Just start tomorrow. You may also find charting your workout progress to be as helpful as tracking your food and emotions in your journal: you can spot patterns, including weak areas where you're prone to skip activity. My patients who chart their activities each week in a journal are the most successful with maintaining a personal program and knowing when to up the ante. For example, if you don't feel 100 percent on a Wednesday, and you look at your journal and see that you haven't moved your body in any significant way since last Wednesday, you know that you need to schedule more activity in the coming days. No one is perfect every day, but as you chart your habits you'll recognize progress at the same time and realize an enormous sense of satisfaction that can be very rewarding and motivating.

- *Don't go home.* Few people like to finish a whole day of work, go home, change clothes, then go to the gym. Once home, we all would prefer to hit the couch and chill out or play with our family. Going home is way too tempting. Work out before work or on your way home. I don't know anyone who has ever gone home, changed clothes, then gone out to exercise. It may well be impossible.

When living an active life is part of your religion—part of who you are—you'll be amazed at what you can do, and how this achievement transfers over to other areas in your life. Your waistline aside, you'll discover that the active life is a Full life.

The Full Challenge: Day 7

I've given you lots of ideas in this chapter for initiating a regular physical-activity program in your life. Remember, this doesn't mean signing up for a marathon or even joining a gym. Today, I want you to take just one small step by considering Phase 1: Planning. Plan your workouts for the next week. Start with one thing you will do today that engages your body in a whole new way. For you, maybe it's walking briskly around your neighborhood. Or maybe you'll want to check out your local yoga studio for beginner group classes. Call a friend and invite her for a hike in some nearby hills. Whatever. The point is that you plan your exercise as seriously as you plan everything else in your life.

Like you planned your cheats, plan the times when you'll move your body enough to break a sweat each day. And remember to base this on your real schedule—factoring in obligations, time commitments, morning and evening agendas, and so on. The two biggest tips to bear in mind: (1) be realistic and (2) be practical. Although I recommended that you aim to exercise for an hour a day, five days a week, don't try to be so ambitious right now if you've been sedentary for a long time. Use the ideas in this chapter to build up to this level one day— one step, one block—at a time.

LISA DOZIER

Age: 45, Height: 5'3"
Starting: Weight: 177.2, Size: 14
Final: Weight: 158.8, Size: 10
Total Lost: 18.4 Pounds and 27"

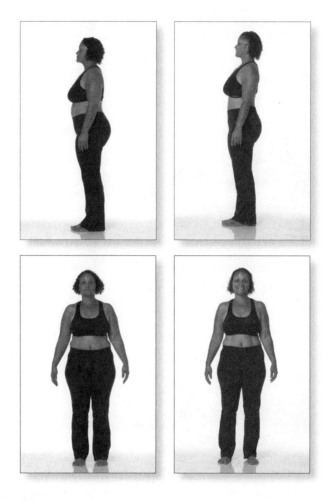

"I have a strong family history of diabetes, and I knew that I had to make a life-style change to remain healthy and active in the years to come. This program finally gave me the diet and fitness routine that I lacked. I now have a better appreciation for the importance of doing both. This is definitely something I can maintain."

CHAPTER EIGHT

Q&A

Following are answers to some frequently asked questions I get from nonsurgical candidates and patients at various stages of their weight-loss journey. In many of the answers you'll find echoes of information I've provided in previous sections of the book, and at times I will refer back to specific pages. If you have a question that is not answered below, just log on to my Website, www.fullbar.com, and ask me there. You'll find other Q&As on the site, too.

Q. What do you think about weight-loss drugs, both over-the-counter and prescription?

A. As noted in Chapter 3, antiobesity drugs do not have an impressive long-term success rate. Besides, if you could take a pill to effortlessly control your weight, don't you think you'd have heard about it by now?

From controlling your debt to your weight, there are no overnight cures. If any of the popular weight-loss solutions were as good as they claim, you'd know about it. Instead, we're more likely to read about serious side effects and unhealthy outcomes that result from the use of medications designed to help with weight loss. Bottom line: there's no free ride, so use caution when considering weight-loss drugs.

This doesn't mean that if you find a weight-loss drug to be effective that you shouldn't experiment with it. Just be sure to do your homework and discuss your options with your doctor, including those that you find in drug stores and don't require a prescription. Be knowledgeable about what you're ingesting and what the potential side effects are; see if you can choose the medications that have a long history and contain natural ingredients. Sometimes people find that taking a drug for weight loss helps them stay mindful of their goal, and there's nothing wrong with that so long as you're not compromising your health to do so. Keep your expectations in check and understand that no matter what supplemental weight-loss drug you choose, the tools in this book will go a long way to enhance any other method you use.

Q. I am about 100 pounds overweight. Does that mean I need surgery to be "normal"?

A. Probably, if your body mass index (BMI) is in the 35 to 39 range (see Chapter 2 for more details about BMI and how to calculate it), and definitely if you are in the 40-plus BMI range. For you, losing weight through traditional methods will be a significant struggle without the surgery. As noted in Chapter 3, the 1992 NIH consensus conference stated that 95 percent of people who try voluntary weight-loss options (programs, behavioral therapy, diet drugs, and so on) will gain their weight back within five years. So statistically, you may need a greater degree of help. Please note that this doesn't mean it's impossible to permanently lose the weight through attention to diet and exercise alone. People have done it in the past, and some will continue to defy the statistics in the future. I'm just saying that the odds are stacked against you once you have at least 100 pounds to lose. Keep in mind that your excess weight likely comes with added health challenges or risks such as diabetes and high blood pressure that can exacerbate metabolic issues and antagonize your best efforts to change your habit and lifestyle.

Q. What do you think about products marketed to increase metabolism? Do they help?

A. There's no shortage of products today marketed to give you the upper hand in revving your metabolism, boosting your energy levels, "burning fat," and "melting pounds." Most of these products contain similar ingredients: stimulants such as caffeine, taurine, guarana, and the like. These can increase your energy level, which can help you to stay focused on, say, your weight-loss goals, but have not been shown to promote a significant durable weight loss. They are not silver bullets for weight loss and should not be considered life-changing metabolic enhancers no matter what the label or advertisement says.

If you choose to include these in your diet, watch out for hidden sugar—the sugar, not the stimulant, may be the reason why you feel so energetic afterward (just before you crash and then seek another sugary carbohydrate to bring you back up again). When you scrutinize the standard energy drink, it's usually loaded with sugar and most cans contain two, sometimes two and a half, servings. This translates to a lot of empty liquid calories that do nothing to enhance your weight-loss efforts or sense of fullness. Be very wary of these drinks. And, as an important medical aside, when using any energy supplement, be careful about any potential side effects. Studies have shown that energy drinks may increase heart rate and blood pressure levels in addition to increasing energy. They may also change how effective medications are. The ingredient taurine, for example, which is an amino acid found in protein-rich foods like meat and fish, can affect heart function and blood pressure.

That said, using such additives as an adjunct to improving your focus and performance in physical activity can sometimes be a rational consideration. But, as I said before, there are no magic bullets. I am against the wanton use and abuse of caffeine, but I allow for some coffee in exchange for activity. If you're working out, feel free to use caffeinated products within reason to help you in your performance—assuming your doctor agrees.

Q. Can you lose weight without exercising?

A. If only I had a dime for every time I'm asked this question. As detailed in Chapter 8, the answer is yes, because physical activity (unless done vigorously like a professional athlete) is a minor component to the economics of weight loss. The unavoidable, critical component is how much you consume.

But don't underestimate the power of exercise in boosting your weight-loss efforts. Even a modest routine that has you moving your body at least three times a week for 30 minutes per session provides a wonderful adjunct to your improved dietary regimen. The health benefits of exercise also cannot be overstated. They range from optimal physiologic functioning to better moods and sound sleep. All of these can factor into your metabolism, motivation, and ability to stay on track. Don't fear physical activity. A sedentary life wastes the opportunities that your body affords you. See Chapter 7 for more details on how to get moving, and establish routines attuned to your likes and dislikes.

Q. I can only handle one change in my life right now related to what and how I eat. Which tool should I start with then?

A. The first tool to start with is mindfulness. Spend a week or two just being aware of what you're eating, why you're eating it, and how full it's making you. Use your journal and the questions in Chapter 5 to record how hungry you are before and after your meals. Mindfulness is key for any subsequent steps you take. If you do nothing else but tune into what and how much you're eating for a week, my guess is you'll automatically begin to make slight shifts in what you're doing to effect radical change in the long run. And it won't feel "radical" in the least.

Once you've spent a week or two just being mindful, begin modulating the volume of your portions (if you haven't naturally done so already). Stay mindful of what fullness means to you. Be aware of what a reasonable portion size is for you so it allows you to be full. And try to incorporate a broad range of food choices into your meals—lean proteins, complex carbohydrates, and healthy fats—so you're not eating loads of one type of food and forgetting the rest. Once you're comfortable engaging this level of mindfulness and control, then frequency of meals and planning meals accordingly will be easier.

Q. Is it possible for a person to overstretch that top 10 percent of the stomach and be doomed forever?

A. If you routinely overeat and are not mindful of the massive volumes you're consuming, you'll soon burn your body out of being able to effectively tell you when to stop eating. Luckily, this isn't a gear you will remain stuck in forever. You can reset your body's fullness center simply by heading back toward sensibly sized meals. Remember, fullness is within all of us.

Q. How does hydration factor into the Full effect? Can drinking water, for example, really fill you up? If so, how much and when should it be taken?

A. Hydration is as essential to weight loss as it is to life. Our bodies need water to function and I recommend that everyone aim to drink a glass of water with every meal. It helps to also drink water as a premeal trick because it can assist you in reaching that non-negotiable full sensation. I cover the hydration factor at length in Chapter 4. Though sodas, fruit juice, and sports drinks can also play into hydration, be careful about drinking too many liquid calories. If you do nothing else but cut back on caloric beverages and stick to plain water (regular or sparkling), you can see a difference on the scale in a relatively short time period.

Q. Should I take vitamins? Which ones?

A. I don't have anything against vitamins, so long as you've discussed them with your doctor and they are considered alongside other medications you may be taking (prescription or over-the-counter). It can be a challenge to get all of our nutrients from food alone today, so vitamins do help in this regard to fill in the blanks. But you won't find me giving specific recommendations on which vitamins to take. My standards are low: Choose a daily multi that you like and can tolerate. You may also choose to add other vitamins to your regimen as well, such as a fish oil supplement and vitamin D. Vitamins alone won't spur weight loss, but they can be a smart addition to any healthy protocol. When you give your body the raw ingredients it needs to carry out its operations maximally, you optimize the body's environment to take care of its metabolism and support its weight-loss physiology.

When considering vitamins specifically marketed to help you burn fat and boost metabolism, the same advice I gave about energy drinks applies: read up on their ingredients and don't be fooled into thinking a pill can dramatically change your metabolism and fat-burning capacity for the better. There are no shortcuts. And sometimes these vitamins can have unintended consequences with regard to their potential side effects, or the complications they may potentially have with other medications you may be taking.

Q. What do you think about detoxes and cleanses? Are they good for weight loss?

A. Theoretically, the point of a detoxification (or cleanse) program is to cleanse your body of elements that have built up and could potentially cause weight gain, low energy, fatigue, headaches, cramps, and so on. Again, *if it really worked it would be on the front page of the newspaper*. Virtually all detox programs involve hydration as a critical component and the addition of supplements that you're buying at a premium. Let me make it clear (again!) that there are no miracles to be found in a bottle. Most of the weight loss that you experience during a detox process can actually be attributed to water loss. There's a reason such programs only last five to ten days. That's the period of acute water weight loss given the dietary changes that are recommended during detox.

I'll also share that as someone who has operated on thousands of GI tracts, colons are not filled with old deposits of food clinging to their walls. Taking cathartics that help you poop a lot will result in weight loss just from the volume of stool excreted. But if you're reading this book, I can pretty much guarantee that's not the weight loss you're looking for. As you resume your normal diet again post-detox, your body will go back to where it was before in terms of weight and how much you're defecating.

If you choose to do a detox, again be careful about which program you decide to use, and discuss this with your doctor. For some people, detox regimens can help reboot your drive to make changes in how you eat, as well as extinguish cravings for certain foods like those high in fat and sugar. They can give you discipline, break some bad habits, motivate you, and jump-start your fat-burning engines. But a detox needn't be extreme. Leave the real "detox" of cleaning up your system of toxins to your kidneys and liver, which is what they are supposed to do, and focus instead on creating your own detox plan by the following tip: skip food products, chemicals, sugar, alcohol, and caffeine, and replace them with organic vegetables, whole grains, and healthy fats . . . and you've got yourself a cleanse that will work with the body.

Q. Is there any single food I should just eliminate entirely from my life?

A. I don't believe in evicting any food that you like from your life. If it's a food that you know can sabotage your weight goals, then just make it part of your cheat prescription and watch your portions. French fries are my weakness. They are my number-one cheat food, and I'm mindful of how much of them I eat.

Q. Which restaurants should I avoid?

A. It's not the restaurant's fault that you're willing to accept massive serving sizes. Just as you shouldn't have to eliminate any single food from your life, you similarly shouldn't have to walk past any restaurant. Immediately upon thinking about controlling your dietary intake, I bet you have an image of what two or three restaurants you frequently patronize that would undermine your efforts. What do you do? You utilize your portion tool first, and add any others that feel appropriate. Have your waiter bring you a box and shove half of your serving into your take-out container. When I'm in a big city, I love to give my extras to the homeless, so I also ask for a to-go fork. They can use the extra calories. You can't. For more about dealing with "toxic environments," see Chapter 6.

Q. I've always been an emotional eater. I eat when I'm bored, tired, stressed, frustrated . . . you name it. What advice can you give me?

A. It's human nature to eat based on emotions. You're already one step ahead of the game just by knowing that you're an emotional eater, though no one is a *hopelessly* emotional eater. Stated another way, you're at a distinct advantage because you are already in touch with your feelings and their association with your lack of food control. That's fantastic. You've already taken the critical, initial first step of being mindful. The best advice I can give you is twofold. First, keeping track of your emotions and your eating habits will be key. This allows you to identify patterns in your emotional eating behavior and be able to plan for them, or at least stay mindful about the fact you're eating based on emotions and do what you can to modulate your volume accordingly. Work to limit impulse eating. Second, have healthy food options and diversions available so when emotions strike and you cannot avoid impulse eating, at least you can choose foods that won't do too much damage. You may even be able to avoid food altogether by engaging in another activity. We tend to nosh on junk food when emotions call, or sit in front of the television and ruminate over our feelings with our mouths moving mindlessly. Change your environment; get up and go for a walk or call a friend. If your mouth needs something to chew on, reach for vegetables or fruit. Take time to tune into your hunger and gauge how hungry you really are. Your emotions may be hungry for resolution, but your stomach may not be hungry for anything at all.

Q. I have a metabolism that's slower than molasses. What can I do?

A. I don't know anyone looking to lose weight who doesn't complain about a slow metabolism. The good news: in the vast majority of cases, there is nothing inherently "wrong" with one's metabolism. In other words, you're not plagued by a dysfunctional metabolism or illness that renders it permanently slow. Metabolic disorders are few and far between, and there's a lot you can do to speed up your metabolism naturally. Two of the most underestimated factors in keeping a metabolism humming are: (1) frequency of meals, and (2) muscle mass.

Eating every three to four hours has its metabolic advantages. Your metabolism needs to stay gassed if it's to operate maximally. When you skip a meal or reduce your calories significantly, your body will go into preservation ("starvation") mode and downshift its metabolism to protect itself. Then, the next time you do eat, your metabolism won't be working as efficiently and can easily send calories into fat cells for storage thinking it won't get another meal anytime soon. As I noted earlier, bodybuilders who try to get their fat mass down to record-low levels eat around the clock. They don't give their bodies any chance to downshift into a slower mode. For you, eating around the clock means having a breakfast within an hour of rising, and then eating something every three to four hours thereafter.

The second important factor is muscle mass. Muscle is a high-maintenance tissue—it requires a lot of energy (calories!) to maintain. Translation: muscle burns calories. In most people, muscle strength peaks at about ages 20 to 30, then gradually decreases. Without strength training, most people experience a 30 percent loss in overall strength by age 70. If you do nothing else but increase your muscle mass, you'll automatically send your metabolism skyrocketing as your body adjusts to having to sustain that muscle mass. And the ideal way to increase your lean muscle mass is to engage in more physical activity and, in particular, weight-bearing activities (strength training) that force your muscles to get stronger. Taking a brisk walk with a pair of three-pound weights in your hands can get you started. Experiment with various gym equipment, or try a group class that involves strength training (yoga, Pilates and mat Pilates, step aerobics, kickboxing). There are a limitless number of options.

Q. How much do hormones factor into the weight-loss equation? I have a feeling my changing hormones are ruining my chances of losing weight.

A. There's no question that changing hormones can antagonize weight loss and maintenance, especially as we age. Remember, every year after age 25, our body's composition begins to shift quite dramatically. We tend to gain fat weight while losing muscle weight, and as a result, our resting metabolism slows down. Lifestyle changes later in life involving kids, work, and hectic schedules also translate to us being less physically active. While hormones do factor into your metabolism, it's not fair to blame all of your weight problems on hormones or think that a magic pill or potion can cure your hormonal challenges and suddenly awaken your metabolism. Certainly genetics and special conditions such as thyroid issues can come into play when we look at weight gain and metabolism, but one factor that we often overlook is muscle mass. Have the hormone conversation with your doctor to rule out any underlying conditions that could be addressed medically, but then take a good look at the habits you keep to build and maintain muscle mass.

And while it's true that in theory a calorie is a calorie, the body responds differently to the source of calories. Eating a doughnut that is loaded with refined sugar and unhealthy fat will cause a spike in insulin, which triggers storage of those calories in fat cells.

Eating a grilled chicken sandwich on whole-grain bread with bell peppers and avocados, on the other hand, doesn't cause such a dramatic spike and requires time and an expenditure of energy to break down its proteins, healthy fats, and complex carbohydrates. In other words, the sandwich will maximize your metabolism while the doughnut will potentially slow it down.

Q. Does it make a difference if I buy organic or not?

A. With so much talk today about organic foods, people can begin to wonder if buying organic makes it easier to lose weight. It doesn't take an advanced degree to know that whole, natural foods are better for you than processed or fast food. But whether or not you spring for the (more expensive) organic varieties won't necessarily make weight loss any quicker or easier. If you focus on real, natural foods, you're probably in the "organic" category already.

Q. How often should I weigh myself?

A. As I pointed out earlier, don't obsess over daily weight fluctuations. Ideally, weigh yourself once every two weeks maximum, at the same time of day, same place, wearing the same clothes (or naked), and on the same scale. If you can't help yourself, have someone hide the scale so you're not checking your weight every time you enter the bathroom. If possible, weigh yourself outside your home, such as at a gym or in a neighbor's house. My patients can only weigh themselves inside my office.

Q. I hate my thighs. Is there anything I can do to just get rid of them and *then* lead a full life?

A. How your body holds weight is mostly genetically determined. Some people have a tendency to gain weight in certain areas over others. For women, the hips and thighs can be problematic; for men, it's their belly. Unfortunately, there's no such thing as "spot-reducing"—focusing on a single area to reduce its size. I've witnessed hundreds of people perform hundreds, if not thousands, of exercises like lunges and squats in a desperate attempt to slim their lower half. But working just one area where you carry your body fat may not help. The way to achieve a leaner anything (belly, legs, thighs, and so on) is to increase your lean muscle tissue *throughout* your body. By working all your muscles, you increase metabolism. So just by revving your metabolism with the tools in this book you'll start looking the way you want to.

Q. How much of my weight is genetically determined? Is any of my fate reversible?

A. Most of my patients are genetically predetermined to be overweight, especially given today's food environment of plenty. But that doesn't mean they cannot use behavioral tactics to lessen the impact of their genes. Behavior still accounts for more of your weight than genes alone. In fact, only 25 percent of your weight is truly determined by your genes. At any time in your life, you can dramatically change your body weight by combining low-calorie eating and physical activity. Even a person whose genetics spell obesity can lead a lean, fit life with the right set of tools and a commitment to modifying his or her behavior around food. It also bears repeating that your metabolism is never written in stone, even if you don't think your genetics are helping you out in this department. Here's something to think about: In one case study performed at Tufts University, researchers found that individuals in their 90s who strength-trained three times a week for eight weeks increased their strength by 300 percent! Imagine what that did to their metabolisms. So to answer your question simply, while genetics do factor into your weight, your overall weight is not all genetically determined and you can, in fact, change your weight—and metabolism—through targeted strategies.

Q. As a woman, I'm scared of bulking up if I do strength training exercises. I'm already big-boned and want to look slimmer, not bigger.

A. Women don't have the same muscle-building capacity as men due to a difference in testosterone, which gives men much greater (20 to 30 times) muscle-building potential. In women, strength training shows up as being lean and toned, not bulky! If you find yourself building more muscles than you like, then just back off on the amount of weight and increase your repetitions. So instead of lifting 20 pounds for two repetitions, lift 10 pounds for three or four repetitions. Speak with a trainer to help you tailor a program for you and your body.

CONCLUSION

GET ON WITH YOUR FULL LIFE

Food is so much more than fuel to survive biologically. It's love. Medicine. Solace. An excuse. Comfort. Pleasure. A friend. A fond memory. A celebration. And it can also be frustration. Politics. Heartache. Agony. Guilt. Pain. Addiction. An adversary. A reminder of failings and misgivings. A worst enemy.

Given this potential basket of drama and emotions that revolve around something so critical to survival, is there any wonder how and why we can develop an unhealthy relationship with food and our weight as a consequence? I can't think of anything else in life that's so essential for living yet can leave us so vulnerable to being abused and manipulated by its power.

Know What Food Means to You

When I gained those 50 pounds during the six years of my surgical residency, food was both a lifeline to get through my days, but also a way of coping with my high-stress environment and the expectations placed on me as a budding surgeon. It was not uncommon for me to start the day with a double-sized bowl of Cocoa Puffs with a whole-milk double latte poured over it plus a glazed doughnut or two on the side. I lived on candy bars and pizza. At the time I was in Oregon, where the first wave of the fancy coffee explosion meant coffee carts were everywhere. And a great pastry was always nearby, too. So my weight climbed and climbed. When I finished my residency, my wife and I had a young child and another on the way. I thought that maybe it was time to be more fit and healthy. The attempts to diet began, but only after I stopped all the failed dieting could I control my weight. This came, though, after some self-awareness.

I realized that I was always looking for the next meal to be my entertainment. In my six demanding and painful years of training, and basically living in the hospital, I had little "fun" to look forward to. Food naturally became my fun. This clearly had to change. I came up with the idea that it was time to get on with my life. Throughout my residency, and through much of medical school, the eating process was mostly about getting a break. Whether it was a rest or another type of break, my eating was a way to stop thinking so hard, working so intensely, or worrying so much. In many ways, my life had been reduced to looking forward to the next candy bar. This was not a recipe for success, but it certainly gave me the false energy and sugar-and-caffeine rush I was addicted to.

So I decided to stop lusting after foods and seeing meals as a source of distraction. When you are honest with yourself about the "value" of meals, then you can figure out what you want them to mean to you. I thought long and hard about the fact that eating distractions had taken over a part of me. I could not tolerate that. The entertainment value of eating and the fun of food were way too important to me. There had to be a better way to live.

I decided to see meals as more about feeding the biological machine and less about keeping me happy and entertained. I work now to teach my patients the same thought process, albeit with a consideration for their limitations and individual needs, and that is my hope for readers. Sometimes, however, we do need to be reminded.

Take, for example, a picnic I once hosted for a group of my patients; by virtue of the fact it was a picnic, the focus was on activities and socializing. At the start of this picnic, I was struck by one of my patients who'd gone back to old habits. He arrived at the picnic, sat down in front of the food spread, and started to eat. He didn't really interact with anyone or even see what kind of activities and distractions we had on hand. He just positioned himself at the food and ate. The fact that he'd been surgically made to eat substantially less food had no effect on his thoughts and actions. Clearly, the habit of food being the focus still held him strongly. When I pointed this out to him, however, he quickly realized his behavior patterns and felt empowered to choose another approach to this setting. Just being made aware of this allowed him to break the cycle and enjoy hanging out and playing games at the picnic—rather than it being all about the food.

Now Get On with Your Life!

When I eat lunch in the middle of my day now, I do the following. I put the meal on the plate—I am very aware of what my portion is made up of and that it is a reasonable serving size. I eat it. Then I go back to work. I spend no time thinking, *Am I full?* I eat, walk away, and then get on with my life. I know, through the science of fullness, that I am guaranteed to be appetite-satisfied about 20 minutes after I eat. It always works out. Now if I just plowed through lunch and kept looking for immediate satisfaction then I would continue packing it in. And I'd feel terrible and stuffed throughout the day. Instead, I rely on my fullness mechanisms to guarantee that I am not going to stomp around like a ravished zombie. (That would not go over well in surgery.) The doctors' lounge is rife with food temptations and indulgences despite the notion that we physicians know better. I remind myself that it's not about feeling stuffed. It's about eating a sensible meal and getting back to what is really important: getting on with life.

This doesn't mean your eating routine will be the same, but however you choose to eat, the experience should be similar: Let your brain be responsible for being satisfied. It will always come through. Give it time. This sounds like common sense. But when you eat a meal, don't you often think, *What more can I have? I'm still hungry. I still have more time. My lunch break is not over for another 15 minutes. What more can I eat?* These are common and constant thoughts, but often they are not at the front of your conscious mind. They are so routine that they are just habits. If there is more food around, then we continue to eat. If there is more time at the meal, we keep on eating. Only in this way could we regularly go out to dinner and eat salad, soup, appetizer, main course, and dessert. This is an obscenely large amount of food. No one is hungry for this volume of food. And after a meal like this (that we all have eaten many times!), we hit the parking lot feeling stuffed and bloated.

The science of this "too full" feeling is simple: we ate too fast and too much without allowing our brain to feel fullness. The meal had nothing to do with what we wanted or needed to eat. We just set ourselves up for eating a "big meal" and prepared ourselves to, as a patient of mine frequently says, "Strap on the feedbag." If you don't wait and allow the nerve and hormone messages time to get to your brain, then you will only realize you are full ("stuffed") when it's too late . . . when you have gone way beyond the regular capacity of your stomach. The stretch is too great. It's not a wonderful feeling. But it's one we have learned to associate with feasts and parties. What is Thanksgiving without this stuffed feeling? Depend on and trust the science of fullness and how you are wired. You will not be disappointed with the results.

Keeping the Family Happy and Healthy in Mind and Body

At this point you may be wondering how to keep everyone else in your family happy as you shift your approach to food and eating. You may ask: How do I talk to my kids about diet and nutrition? How do I talk to a child who enjoys video games more than playing outside and is showing signs of becoming overweight?

These are all important questions. People are always wondering how they can deal with nutrition, health, and weight issues with their children. The fear is that you may affect their self-esteem, make them "feel fat," or trigger an eating disorder. Clearly, all of us would do anything in our power to avoid these problems, which are very real in today's culture. According to the Centers for Disease Control and Prevention, a full third of America's children are overweight, and 17 percent are clinically obese, a rate that has more than tripled since 1976. Those figures may be alarming, yet equally disturbing are the numbers of children, girls in particular, who risk their health in the other direction, in the vain pursuit of thinness. In a 2002 survey of 81,247 Minnesota high-school students published in the *Journal of Adolescent Health*, more than half of the girls reported engaging in some form of disordered behavior while trying to lose weight: fasting, popping diet pills, smoking, vomiting, abusing laxatives, or binge eating.

As a parent, you can feel stuck, worrying about the perils of both obesity and anorexia. What's more, we may pay more attention to our daughters than our sons. According to a study of preschool girls published in the journal *Pediatrics* in 2001, those whose mothers expressed "higher concern" over their daughters' weights not only reported more negative body images than their peers but also perceived themselves as less smart and less physically capable (paternal "concern" was associated only with the latter). The effect was independent of the child's actual size. A 2003 analysis of the National Health and Nutrition Examination Survey, meanwhile, showed that mothers were three times as likely to notice excess weight in daughters as in sons, even though the boys were more likely to be large.

No parent can opt out of talking about food and weight. Avoiding conversations about food, health, and body image would be impossible. I wish all of my fellow parents would make it a goal to establish a healthy, ongoing dialogue about food and weight with their children—regardless of their size and sex. Pardon me for sounding preachy when it comes to dispensing parenting advice, but many parents have found the ideas I'm about to share incredibly helpful and enlightening. So do what you want with the following information—if some of this resonates with you, great. If not, move on and don't look back.

To start, let me share what I believe to be the four chief areas in a child's life that, as parents, we hope they live up to our expectations. Virtually all of us want kids to:

- Be intellectually engaged. Study, read, think, have an active and inquisitive mind, and do as well as they can in school.

- Be involved in the community. Show an appreciation and respect for others, whether that entails just friends or higher levels of community participation such as volunteer work, religious groups, clubs, and so on.

- Be emotionally engaged. Communicate well, with access to their feelings and the ability to talk about them to you and others they trust. How your children communicate is a huge part of who they are and how people perceive and treat them.

- Be vigorous and actively engaged in life. Make physical activity a part of daily life and explore what the body is capable of: *movement.*

Now I ask you, how can any of these goals be achieved without a strong, healthy body supporting them in these pursuits? None of the above vision we have for our children could be possible unless they have a healthy personal relationship with their bodies. As they mature into thoughtful, productive adults, they need to develop healthy behaviors around food and the act of eating. And that's primarily accomplished with your help in guiding them through the inevitable challenges they may face. By taking control of your own eating life with the ideas in this book, you can then set a great example for your children that they will carry for the rest of their lives.

Lead by Example

Pardon the dramatic examples, but consider the following: You can't just tell your kids to go to church or synagogue; you must go with them. You don't demand that your kids limit their TV viewing; you limit TV viewing as a family. You don't spout out profanities and demand that your kids only use clean language. You don't laze around the couch wearing sweat-stained shirts and encourage your kids to shower regularly. By subscribing to the sensible eating guidelines outlined in this book, you will be inspiring everyone in your life to similarly embrace moderation. Your goal is to be thoughtful without being oppressive in dietary choices and to be engaged in healthful eating without misery, sacrifice and pain.

Create an environment that encourages a sound diet and regular exercise. Fill your house with the right foods, and eliminate those things that no one should be eating on a regular basis. If you are too busy to cook for your family and fast food is a way of life, don't think your kids will understand any other way of eating. Eating well takes mindfulness and some work, as you know, so require the same of your kids. As I mentioned earlier, see if you can set aside certain days of the week when you eat dinner as a family. Family meals around a table are among the most powerful teachers of self-control; they teach that the appetite of the moment is not the sole determinant of one's behavior. Even better: cook as a family and then sit together over a shared meal. Don't allow electronic distractions to accompany those meals, such as cell phones and hand-held devices that will steal your kids' minds away from the full eating experience. Indulgences should be allowed in your kids the same way they are allowed for you—as planned cheats in an otherwise reasonable dietary regimen.

As you transition to a healthier lifestyle, you may be surprised to find your entire family adapting. There are times when family members, especially kids, can be enablers with junk food. And for whatever reason, you may not want to restrict all of that from them. So what else can you do to prevent yourself from falling for it? Do what I do: buy foods that they love but which you hate. For example, I buy my kids treats that contain coconut or marshmallows because I don't enjoy those—but my kids do.

> If you live with people who insist on having junk food available, make it as inaccessible to you as possible. This may mean relegating junk food to high shelves, hiding it behind other essentials so it's not so visible, and double-bagging foods in the freezer and refrigerator that you find irresistible, such as ice cream or cheese. Keep a package of gum or Listerine strips in a kitchen drawer to pop into your mouth if something in the kitchen tickles your salivary glands and you know it's not an appropriate time to indulge.

Stress Health and Balance, Not Weight

My second piece of advice is to remember that it's not about weight; it's about health and balance. I never allow my kids to be talked about in terms of controlling their weight. It's a recipe for having a distorted perspective that may result in a lifetime of maladaptive eating. If it's all about controlling your weight, then all that matters is minimizing calories, which is a recipe for potentially dangerous eating behaviors in the future. Use the words *healthy, feeling good,* and *being fit.* Never make it about being thin or skinny.

Eliminate unrealistic images from your life as much as possible. As my kids started to move into what I call the "aware years" (eight to ten), they began to comment on how actresses and models looked on TV shows and magazines. As a family, my wife and I worked to limit their exposure to such images. We canceled subscriptions to air-brushed, digitally enhanced magazines and reduced our viewing of shows that have similarly unrealistic images or that convey unhealthy messages. Watch your own commentary on body image dissatisfaction and weight control. If Mom and Dad are always talking about calories, restrictions, feeling fat, how they look, and so on, then that becomes as important to your kids.

Be aware of how your children have accepted weight conversation and body-image issues into their life already, and address them head-on. In Denver, I recently gave a lecture to middle-school parents and was astonished to find that parents of seventh-grade girls were reporting how much their daughters complained about their body and weight. According to these parents, it's "cool" to complain about weight and fat. And in order to feel part of the group, their daughters had to express such dissatisfaction about their appearance. This is the sad reality of our world today.

I know it's been said a million times, but you have to lead by example. Again, it's not about losing weight. It's about using the body that you've been given and making the most of it. Having vigorous activity in daily life is important to you, and you should require it of your children, too. Make them aware of heart health and the effects of exercise at the exclusion of talking about the exercise benefits in terms of their weight. Having that kind of awareness—the importance of moving the body through space—will give them a lifetime of health and, as an offshoot, potentially help them control their weight. This should not feel punishing, and it's not about shoving them out the door and telling them to go play outside.

Find out what they like and create a world that allows them to participate in those activities. Engage them in activities that they enjoy. It's perfectly fine to discover this through trial and error, making sure they have the resources to do what they love. You'll be amazed at how many kids want to be active but don't know what to do. And it wouldn't be terrible if you were both active together. Make it a family way of living. On Saturday morning, for instance, go on a family walk together. On Sunday evening, play Frisbee in the backyard. It's a great time to have unpressured discussions about what life is really like. You're both sweating on a walk or playing in the yard, messing up your hair, and wearing sweaty clothes. This may be the ideal moment to talk about schoolwork, friends, happiness, or what's bothering your kids.

Not every kid is going to be a weekend soccer superstar and be able to tolerate weekday practices. I like going to the gym for physical and mental health. My kids have always seen me sweaty after a morning at the gym and know that dad "needs to go or he gets grumpy." My son tried team sports but they weren't the thing for him. Like me, he enjoys going to the gym and hitting the weight machines after spending time on the treadmill. It's an efficient use of his time and keeps him active without having to force himself to participate in the organized sports world that proved not fun for him. Though he's an accomplished musician, being a talented guitarist does not exclude him from being active.

Get Help When Necessary

It's really important that you stay attuned to your kids' self-image and feelings. You want them to live as full a life as possible, and not enter a self-defeating cycle of punishment and guilt that constantly revolves around weight issues and unhappiness about one's appearance.

When your kids are complaining about their weight, or perhaps becoming overweight, I recommend discussing this with their pediatrician and making an appointment for an assessment. Your pediatrician is a neutral third party and can help defuse some of the emotions you may be harboring about discussing these sensitive issues with your child. If you're not comfortable having this kind of conversation with your pediatrician, change pediatricians. And if there really is an imbalance in your child's diet and activity levels, I encourage you to obtain a referral to a qualified nutritionist or registered dietitian who has been referred by your pediatrician. This is a great opportunity to start your child out with an objective perspective on what they need to do and how they need to eat.

I'm not blindly pawning off your parental responsibilities on psychological and dietary experts; rather, I'm trying to make it clear that I don't want your child to ever feel you're actively judging what they do or how they eat because that will never turn out well. Use these neutral resources to your benefit. Also, while you're in front of these experts with your child, establish ground rules as to how you can engage your kids in this ongoing discussion. What help are you allowed to give and how comfortable is your child with your support? You should not be the food and activity police. You are to support the rules given by the professionals. Any other way of behaving will result in an endless struggle of pain and strife between you and your child. This is the one time you need to get a professional involved.

How Dare You!

As a physician I always find that I have to blindly accept my patients' behaviors and attitudes in order to objectively shepherd them through their medical experience. It's not my job to judge, and I've been trained specifically to "take all comers" when they are trusting me to help them with their health. But I feel like I have to come clean and let you into a little bit of reality with regard to setting limitations. I've had to share this perspective more than once with a particularly difficult patient or two.

I love all of my patients dearly, but if I had to pinpoint the ones who give me my greatest challenges, it's those who have had all the advantages of the surgery and my bariatric program but have worked very hard to fail in their weight-loss pursuits.

On my worst days, or when I think it's most beneficial to these patients, I will let them know my feelings and saddle them with the real perspective of my frustration. I might say, "How dare you put your health and life at risk and drag your family through surgery and recovery only to reach this disappointing juncture! How dare you not fulfill this, violating the trust that your family put in you!"

I know this rant may seem overly paternalistic, and maybe even nasty or insensitive, but isn't it the hard truth? Don't my patients have an obligation to fulfill their commitment to themselves and their families?

On the (very) rare occasion that I have to deliver this lecture, it's usually met with a lot of tears and "I'm sorry." I remind them that they shouldn't be apologizing to me. They should be sorry for what they've put their family through and instigate the changes immediately that everyone (including themselves) expected. I tell them to become the person they promised to be and get over their fear of success. Because that's what it really boils down to: a fear of success. They can begin the process seriously at any time. So can you.

Tough Love

Clearly, when you bought this book, you were not making quite the same level of commitment as my patients do when they choose to undergo a radical surgical procedure. You opened this book because you were curious to learn about a potentially new way to lose weight. The only commitment you had to make was dishing out the dollars to purchase the book and then take the time to read it. You may think that this is not a heroic or even a very serious accomplishment, but I wholeheartedly disagree. Almost everyone reading this has spent many years or a lifetime engaged in the struggle to control their weight. The effect on your person, body, psyche, and self-esteem, has been monumental. And don't think for a moment that your family and friends haven't been through the struggle with you. When your happiness is tied to the fit of your jeans or to your morning weigh-in, everyone around you is affected.

When you change the way you act toward your spouse or loved ones because of whether or not you feel attractive or good about yourself—or because you think you've failed in the weight-loss arena—it has an indelible impact on your family and friends. Regardless of how much weight you think you have to lose, think about how much your waistline influences how you interact with people and how you feel about yourself. In this regard, you're not too different from my patients. Your loved ones have always been and continue to be an integral part of your weight-loss struggle, whether you mean for it to be or not. Like I say to my patients, how dare you put them through that agony without realizing the effects it has on them and their world?

How dare you not be sensitive to their concern and disappointment when you make them part of your concern and sadness? It's really not that much different than my patients who violate the rules and tools that have been given to them to have success, health, and happiness. It's a whole different battle when it's not just you against the scale. But in reality, it's you and your family's happiness and health engaged in the struggle. Don't think for a moment that your friends, family, co-workers, job productivity, and so much else is not participating in the struggle with you. Nothing about you exists in the vacuum, especially when it affects how you feel about yourself. The constant repetition of hope, short-term gain, and ultimate failure is truly injurious not just to you, but to all parts of your life, including your loved ones. You know this is true.

The diet industry is so powerful that it can suck my own patients back into its vortex from time to time. They will come back to me years after their surgery and present a complex recounting of how they are "succeeding." They dive into an enthusiastic conversation about how they've taken up the torch again for [diet X], or reapplied the rules of the [Y] diet, or started to follow the personal prescriptions of their personal trainer. Case in point: Someone recently told me how he always follows the [very popular] diet when he needs to lose weight because it has worked so well for him the last 15 times he's done it. It's the "only thing" that helps him drop the pounds. I countered that it may have worked once—but it has failed 15 times.

It must be human nature to return to thinking that diets work, which compels people to go back to a certain diet and go in circles all over again. Once more, they are taking on the unrealistic responsibility of adhering to an overly complex, overly demanding regimen in the face of my simple recommendations for durable and significant weight loss.

The Power of Fullness

My patients sleep through the surgery while I do all of the work. But they are responsible from that point forward—they have to do the work for the next 20, 30, 40, 50 years. How do people who have had many years of failed weight loss succeed after the surgery? Here's a hint: It is not the surgery. Rather, it's their ability to succeed at feeling full with a small meal. The power of fullness is what's most important in their lives.

My patients have been to a world that most of you have only visited in your worst dreams. Having a BMI of 35-plus is very hard to live with. So they are willing to make strong and ironclad commitments to "never go there again." They have perspective and realize the gift of fullness. They actively court it at every turn. Trust me, they know that they could drink those rich, caramel, calorie-laden "domed drinks" at their local coffee shop. But such food would not make them full and would result in too many empty calories. They know it is all about "being full." That's what keeps them away from the rich drinks. When they are full, it's no longer about control. It's about truly not desiring the junk.

Remember, food holds no power over you when you are full.

Choice Is Also Power

Take the steps to constantly keep hunger out of your life. Make the choice to be successful. Be aware that it is much easier to fail and many of us are used to failing. It is often the path of least resistance —it comes easily to many people and they are comfortable with failure. It is no longer an option to fail when you decide that you want to get on with your life. Isn't thinking about weight issues a bit boring? Don't you have better things to do? I know that you do. You owe it to yourself, your family, and your world.

Most people are so used to the constant internal dialogue about their weight, diet, and activity considerations that they really don't know of any other way to be. When you go to a coffee shop or café, the question of "What do I want?" is trumped by the act of staring at the overhead board of food and coffee choices and thinking, *What's not going to make me fat?* And, this is repeated at every meal and eating opportunity—four to six times per day. For life. Shouldn't there be more to living? Aren't there better uses for our energy? Wouldn't it be better to execute a simple plan utilizing my simple tools than to make such constant negotiations and accounting in this omnipresent part of our lives?

Remember, the ultimate weapon you have that separates you from all other species is your amazingly powerful brain. So use the conscious and primitive parts of your brain to your ultimate advantage. Work to organize your world for your success. Make conscious food decisions. Plan your meals. Prepare ahead of time. Plan your cheats. Make time and plan for activities that get your body moving. Keep your tools in mind at all times. Memorize them and apply as many to your life as you can, when you can. These are your conscious brain's activities.

Then, use your primitive brain, the part of your brain that has strong needs that must be satisfied or will take over your life. Understand that your brain is in constant search of satisfaction. It has a quest for it! So work to keep it satisfied. The "narcotic" of fullness is your ultimate weapon against your primitive self. Stay full and you will be able to move on in your life. When full, your primitive brain is happy and will leave you alone to get on with your life. It always works. I can make it work through surgery. You can make it work through the tools in this book. It is something you can depend on. It will make all of the difference. I rest my reputation on it.

The big question is: "What will you do now that you are full?"

I believe that you will think of something amazing to do.

I have faith in you.

Appendix A:

BODY MASS INDEX TABLE

Body Mass Index Table

Body Weight (pounds)

Height (inches)	Normal						Overweight					Obese										Extreme Obesity															
BMI	19	20	21	22	23	24	25	26	27	28	29	30	31	32	33	34	35	36	37	38	39	40	41	42	43	44	45	46	47	48	49	50	51	52	53	54
58	91	96	100	105	110	115	119	124	129	134	138	143	148	153	158	162	167	172	177	181	186	191	196	201	205	210	215	220	224	229	234	239	244	248	253	258
59	94	99	104	109	114	119	124	128	133	138	143	148	153	158	163	168	173	178	183	188	193	198	203	208	212	217	222	227	232	237	242	247	252	257	262	267
60	97	102	107	112	118	123	128	133	138	143	148	153	158	163	168	174	179	184	189	194	199	204	209	215	220	225	230	235	240	245	250	255	261	266	271	276
61	100	106	111	116	122	127	132	137	143	148	153	158	164	169	174	180	185	190	195	201	206	211	217	222	227	232	238	243	248	254	259	264	269	275	280	285
62	104	109	115	120	126	131	136	142	147	153	158	164	169	175	180	186	191	196	202	207	213	218	224	229	235	240	246	251	256	262	267	273	278	284	289	295
63	107	113	118	124	130	135	141	146	152	158	163	169	175	180	186	191	197	203	208	214	220	225	231	237	242	248	254	259	265	270	278	282	287	293	299	304
64	110	116	122	128	134	140	145	151	157	163	169	174	180	186	192	197	204	209	215	221	227	232	238	244	250	256	262	267	273	279	285	291	296	302	308	314
65	114	120	126	132	138	144	150	156	162	168	174	180	186	192	198	204	210	216	222	228	234	240	246	252	258	264	270	276	282	288	294	300	306	312	318	324
66	118	124	130	136	142	148	155	161	167	173	179	186	192	198	204	210	216	223	229	235	241	247	253	260	266	272	278	284	291	297	303	309	315	322	328	334
67	121	127	134	140	146	153	159	166	172	178	185	191	198	204	211	217	223	230	236	242	249	255	261	268	274	280	287	293	299	306	312	319	325	331	338	344
68	125	131	138	144	151	158	164	171	177	184	190	197	203	210	216	223	230	236	243	249	256	262	269	276	282	289	295	302	308	315	322	328	335	341	348	354
69	128	135	142	149	155	162	169	176	182	189	196	203	209	216	223	230	236	243	250	257	263	270	277	284	291	297	304	311	318	324	331	338	345	351	358	365
70	132	139	146	153	160	167	174	181	188	195	202	209	216	222	229	236	243	250	257	264	271	278	285	292	299	306	313	320	327	334	341	348	355	362	369	376
71	136	143	150	157	165	172	179	186	193	200	208	215	222	229	236	243	250	257	265	272	279	286	293	301	308	315	322	329	338	343	351	358	365	372	379	386
72	140	147	154	162	169	177	184	191	199	206	213	221	228	235	242	250	258	265	272	279	287	294	302	309	316	324	331	338	346	353	361	368	375	383	390	397
73	144	151	159	166	174	182	189	197	204	212	219	227	235	242	250	257	265	272	280	288	295	302	310	318	325	333	340	348	355	363	371	379	386	393	401	408
74	148	155	163	171	179	186	194	202	210	218	225	233	241	249	256	264	272	280	287	295	303	311	319	328	334	342	350	358	365	373	381	389	396	404	412	420
75	152	160	168	176	184	192	200	208	216	224	232	240	248	256	264	272	279	287	295	303	311	319	327	335	343	351	359	367	375	383	391	399	407	415	423	431
76	156	164	172	180	189	197	205	213	221	230	238	246	254	263	271	279	287	295	304	312	320	328	336	344	353	361	369	377	385	394	402	410	418	426	435	443

Appendix B:

A PHASED APPROACH TO WEIGHT LOSS

By now I hope that you've incorporated (or at least thought about) the tools I've been describing, especially with regard to portion control and mindful eating. Don't hesitate to reread chapters to remind yourself how to allocate your meals and portions properly, handle cheats, and routinely check in with your hunger levels. Remember, try to avoid feeling like a stuffed 10 and instead, sense a comfortable 5.

There are two options for working your way through *The Full Diet:*

1. Go through my Induction Phase for a total of four weeks using the step-by-step instructions below. Then, shift to the Continuing Success Phase for as long as you need to reach your ideal weight. Caution: If you have been sedentary for a long time and you are significantly overweight (your BMI puts you in the upper end of the overweight category or you are obese), then I suggest consulting with your doctor before attempting this Induction. It would be wise for you to ease your way into a new diet and fitness regimen given your individual health circumstances.

2. Simply follow the steps in the Continuing Success Phase if the Induction Phase looks too limiting

(or too intimidating). You will lose just as much weight, but it will take a little longer because you're consuming more food on a daily basis.

When choosing which option to try, there are a number of considerations to take into account. You have to look at your life right now, and decide what you have the time and energy for. You also need to factor in any unique health challenges, which can include the fact that you're severely overweight and out of physical shape. If you're in decent shape but feeling really busy and stressed out, start with the Continuing Success Phase. This will give you a better chance of keeping with the program. Also, for those who are already engaged in an exercise program and who need more calories to keep up with their routines, the Continuing Success protocol may be more realistic for you. If your biggest goal and clearest focus right now is to lose weight and lose it fast, you'll find the Induction Phase to be a more appealing place to start. Most of the people I take through *The Full Diet* program— and success stories you've met throughout the book—go through the Induction Phase. As I said before, this phase can really help you accelerate your journey. It quickly sets the tone for your new lifestyle habits, and it helps you get rid of certain cravings and bad eating behaviors. But be realistic; if you can't stick to the Induction, don't do it. Failure can quickly discourage you. So you decide! For additional advice tailored to your needs, ask your doctor.

Induction Phase:

- *Breakfast:* Full Shake (see page 87) + 1 multivitamin
- *Morning Snack:* Piece of fruit with yogurt or cottage cheese. Choose from any of the snack options on page 249–251 or in Appendix D. Drink a 16-ounce glass of water.
- *Lunch:* Full Shake (see page 87) + piece of fruit

- *Afternoon Snack:* 16-ounce glass of water + large supplement bar (look for one with 4 to 5 grams fiber, 5 to 6 grams of protein, and less than 200 calories)

- *Dinner:* Reasonable Dinner (any listed in Appendix C)

- *Exercise:* One hour a day for five days a week (see Chapter 7; some people will need to build up to this amount of time)

- *Liquid Intake:* All liquid intake should be no calorie. Water is best. Coffee is acceptable but only two cups per day with no-calorie sweeteners, skim milk, soy milk, or almond milk. No lattes.

- *Cheat:* Two cheats allowed per week but must be planned 24 hours in advance (see Chapter 6 for details)

Continuing Success Phase:

- *Breakfast:* Full Shake (see page 87) + 1 multivitamin

- *Morning Snack:* 16-ounce glass of water + any snack from the list on page 249–251 or in Appendix D

- *Lunch:* Reasonable Lunch (any listed in Appendix C) + premeal snack (see Chapter 4 for details)

- *Afternoon Snack:* 16-ounce glass of water + any snack from the list on page 249-251 or in Appendix D

- *Dinner:* Reasonable Dinner (any listed in Appendix C) + premeal snack (see Chapter 4 for details)

- *Exercise:* One hour a day for five days a week (see Chapter 7; some people will need to build up to this amount of time)

- *Liquid Intake:* All liquid intake should be no calorie. Water is best. Coffee is acceptable but only two cups per day with no-calorie sweeteners, skim milk, soy milk, or almond milk. No lattes.

- *Cheat:* Two cheats allowed per week but must be planned 24 hours in advance (see Chapter 6 for details)

Remember, it's up to you whether you want to start with the stricter Induction Phase or not. If you don't enjoy shakes, however, then you may just want to follow the Continuing Success Phase. In the Induction Phase, you need to stick to just what I've outlined above. However, if you're doing the Continuing Success Phase, the shake for breakfast is simply a suggestion. You can feel free to substitute another common-sense meal that follows the specifications I outlined in Chapter 5. For example, you can enjoy two hard-boiled eggs with salsa and a slice of whole-grain bread, or a bowl of high-fiber cereal, or a cup of yogurt with berries on top. Like I've been saying, this is common sense. A stack of pancakes dripping in syrup, a large white bagel with full-fat cream cheese, a greasy ham and eggs plate, or a bowl of full-fat granola with whole milk should not be options.

And don't forget about portion control! I cannot reiterate the importance of this enough. I encourage you to reread Chapter 5 for explicit details on this critical tool.

Appendix C:

THE FULL DIET MEAL
IDEAS AND RECIPES

Still need me to spoon-feed you meal ideas? In this appendix you'll find a month's worth of lunch ideas and a month's worth of dinner ideas. Most of the lunches are easy to assemble and require little to no cooking; in some instances, such as grilled salmon, you can find these foods already prepared for you at the grocery store—just be sure it hasn't been "processed" in any way with too much sauce or additives. Also, avoid fried versions of the foods listed below. Seek "homemade" versions. If a lunch does require any cooking, simply follow the cooking instructions on the package, and note that most of these dishes can be cooked in the microwave. I tried to make this as easy as possible. You'll find recipes for all the dinner ideas following the weekly meal plans below. And remember, always stick to a single serving. See package information for any prepared foods and refer to page 121 to refresh your memory of what constitutes a single serving for nonprepared foods.

One Month of Lunch and Dinner Ideas

With any of the lunches listed below, feel free to add additional spices to make it more flavorful. Spices add minimal calories, and they're a great way to personalize any dish. Also note that any item marked with an asterisk (*) refers to a particular brand that you'll find at any large supermarket chain. I chose to list some brands because I've found them to be high quality and good for my patients' weight-loss efforts. If no brand is listed (or you can't find the listed brand in your supermarket), just find a brand that suits your tastes and meets the general rules you're trying to follow in terms of quality ingredients.

At the deli counter, choose low-sodium cuts of meat where available. Throughout the menu plan, whenever you see a side salad, I've listed 1 cup of lettuce/greens. This is just a base—feel free to add as much lettuce and as many raw vegetables as you'd like, and choose low-fat or fat-free dressings. You can also add a serving of fruit to any meal if you'd like. Remember, these meal ideas are meant to be examples. You can use the guidelines in this book to create your own, or to improvise where necessary if any of these meals don't appeal to you. *The Full Diet* is about choice!

WEEK 1

SUNDAY

Lunch: open-face sandwich using ½ whole-wheat English muffin, BOCA Burger*, large lettuce leaf, tomato + side of carrot and cucumber slices

Dinner: Summer Jambalaya + 1 cup mixed green salad with low-fat dressing

MONDAY

Lunch: sandwich using whole-wheat mini bagel, light The Laughing Cow cheese,* smoked salmon, lettuce, tomato, and pickle wedges

Dinner: Fish Tacos with salsa

TUESDAY

Lunch: salad using canned salmon, cottage cheese, raspberry vinaigrette, sliced mushrooms + side dish of cherry tomatoes and sliced bell pepper rings

Dinner: Lettuce Wraps + cooked asparagus

WEDNESDAY

Lunch: sandwich using light Flatout Flatbread*, bell peppers, grilled chicken (frozen, partially cooked), and salsa + 1 cup mixed green salad with low-fat dressing

Dinner: Sautéed Pork Chops with Apples + ½ cup steamed broccoli and cauliflower

THURSDAY

Lunch: shrimp cocktail with a squeeze of lemon and 1 tablespoon cocktail sauce + sliced mango

Dinner: Buffalo Chicken Salad

FRIDAY

Lunch: sandwich using whole-wheat mini pita, low-sodium deli roast beef, tomato slices, Mini Babybel Light cheese* + sliced carrots and celery sticks

Dinner: Black Bean Pita Burgers + sliced raw vegetables of choice

SATURDAY

Lunch: rotisserie chicken + roasted veggies

Dinner: Spicy Tuna Wrap

WEEK 2

SUNDAY

Lunch: salad of 2 egg whites boiled, 1 ounce low-fat cheese, 1 ounce low-sodium deli ham, and 1 cup lettuce topped with raw broccoli, tomato slices, and low-fat ranch dressing

Dinner: Crab Cake Burgers + ½ cup cooked green beans

MONDAY

Lunch: veggie quesadilla made with small whole-wheat tortilla, low-fat cheese, grilled onions, bell peppers, salsa, and shredded lettuce (grill or microwave)

Dinner: Greek Stuffed Peppers + 1 cup mixed green salad with low-fat dressing

TUESDAY

Lunch: salad using shredded or chopped grilled chicken (frozen, partially cooked), sliced plum, fat-free mayo, tarragon, 1 teaspoon sliced almonds on bed of lettuce and sliced tomatoes

Dinner: Curried Chicken + sautéed bell peppers, onions, and mushrooms

WEDNESDAY

Lunch: open-face sandwiches using two Wasa crackers,* cucumber slices, Mini Babybel Light cheese*, deli turkey + 1 cup green salad with cherry tomatoes and low-fat dressing

Dinner: California Chicken Dinner Salad

THURSDAY

Lunch: open-face sandwich using ½ whole-wheat English muffin and tuna mixed with chopped celery, topped with tomato slice, avocado, and lettuce leaf

Dinner: Mini Pizza + tossed spinach and tomato salad with low-fat dressing

FRIDAY

Lunch: salad using canned artichoke hearts, tomatoes, and cottage cheese on bed of lettuce with low-fat or fat-free Italian dressing

Dinner: Open-Face Bagel Melt + sautéed eggplant and tomatoes

SATURDAY

Lunch: salad using white beans, shredded or chopped chicken (frozen, partially cooked), cilantro, and garlic powder

Dinner: Kabobs + 1 cup mixed green salad with low-fat dressing

WEEK 3

SUNDAY

Lunch: rice bowl with brown rice, shredded carrots, broccoli, tuna, and teriyaki sauce

Dinner: White Bean Chicken Chili + sliced raw vegetables

MONDAY

Lunch: sandwich using light Flatout Flatbread,* low-sodium deli turkey, fat-free mayo, 1 tablespoon sun-dried tomatoes, and avocado

Dinner: Chicken Berry Salad

TUESDAY

Lunch: mini whole-wheat pita bread, hummus, cucumbers, tomatoes, feta cheese, and Greek olives

Dinner: Southwest Turkey Bake + 1 cup mixed green salad with low-fat dressing

WEDNESDAY

Lunch: precooked turkey burger with tomato sauce with ½ cup cooked zucchini, topped with part-skim shredded mozzarella cheese (grill or microwave)

Dinner: Beef Broccoli Salad

THURSDAY

Lunch: salad of 3 boiled eggs, 2 tablespoons fat-free mayo, and chopped celery on 1 slice whole-wheat bread + sliced raw vegetables

Dinner: Chicken Parmesan + ½ cup cooked yellow squash/zucchini

FRIDAY

Lunch: precooked chicken sausage, brown rice, peppers, onions, and broccoli (grill or microwave)

Dinner: sandwich using Pulled Pork with Caramelized Onions + 1 cup mixed green salad with low-fat dressing

SATURDAY

Lunch: precooked chicken breast topped with portabella mushroom, spinach, feta cheese, and garlic powder (to taste) on ½ whole-wheat bun

Dinner: Asparagus & Salmon Spring Rolls + ½ cup cooked green beans

WEEK 4

SUNDAY

Lunch: 1 cup vegetable soup + ½ whole-wheat pita stuffed with low-sodium deli turkey, lettuce, and tomato

Dinner: Slow-Cooker Pot Roast + 1 cup mixed green salad with low-fat dressing

MONDAY

Lunch: open-face sandwiches with two Wasa crackers,* canned tuna, sliced celery, light Italian dressing + cut raw vegetables

Dinner: Almond & Lemon–Crusted Fish with Spinach

TUESDAY

Lunch: precooked turkey burger with slice of low-fat cheese on ½ whole-wheat bun + sautéed spinach with garlic.

Dinner: Meatball Marinara + 1 cup mixed green salad with low-fat dressing

WEDNESDAY

Lunch: refried beans, ground beef, salsa, and lettuce in a small whole-wheat tortilla

Dinner: Chicken with Caribbean Salsa + 1 cup mixed green salad with low-fat dressing

THURSDAY

Lunch: salad using shrimp cocktail, peas, tomatoes, feta cheese, and red-wine vinegar

Dinner: Mediterranean Baked Fish + steamed broccoli

FRIDAY

Lunch: precooked chicken breast topped with ricotta cheese, pasta sauce, and spinach (grill or microwave)

Dinner: Tacos

SATURDAY

Lunch: sandwich using light Flatout Flatbread*, precooked grilled tilapia and cilantro (grill or microwave) + 1 cup mixed green salad with low-fat dressing

Dinner: Chicken Tortilla Soup + 1 cup mixed green salad with low-fat dressing

The Full Diet Recipes

These recipes were created by two registered dieticians; Jessica Crandall, R.D., C.D.E and Susan Drake, M.S., R.D.

ALMOND & LEMON–CRUSTED FISH WITH SPINACH

Makes 4 servings

Cooking spray
Zest and juice of 1 lemon, divided
½ cup sliced almonds, coarsely chopped
1 tablespoon finely chopped fresh dill or 1 teaspoon dried
1 tablespoon plus 2 teaspoons extra-virgin olive oil, divided
1 teaspoon kosher salt, divided
⅛ teaspoon black pepper
1¼ pounds pacific cod or halibut, cut into 4 portions
4 teaspoons Dijon mustard
2 cloves garlic, slivered
1 pound baby spinach
Lemon wedges for garnish

Preheat oven to 400 degrees. Coat a rimmed baking sheet with cooking spray. In a small bowl, combine lemon zest, almonds, dill, 1 tablespoon oil, ½ teaspoon salt, and pepper. Place fish on the prepared baking sheet and spread each portion with 1 teaspoon mustard. Divide the almond mixture among the portions, pressing it onto the mustard. Bake the fish until opaque in the center, about 7 to 9 minutes, depending on thickness.

Meanwhile, heat the remaining 2 teaspoons oil in a skillet over medium heat. Add garlic and cook, stirring, until fragrant but not brown, about 30 seconds. Stir in spinach, lemon juice, and the remaining ½-teaspoon salt and season with pepper. Cook, stirring often, until the spinach is just wilted, about 2 to 4 minutes. Serve fish with spinach and lemon wedges.

ASPARAGUS & SALMON SPRING ROLLS

Makes 6 servings

Spring Rolls:*
24 thick asparagus spears
Two 3- to 4-ounce packages smoked wild salmon
Twelve 8-inch rice-paper wrappers
1 ripe avocado, cut into 24 slices
1 cup shredded carrot
½ cup chopped fresh basil
½ cup chopped fresh mint

Dipping Sauce:
⅓ cup reduced-sodium soy sauce
2 tablespoons orange juice
2 tablespoons lemon juice
2 tablespoons mirin
¼ teaspoon crushed red pepper, or more to taste

To prepare spring rolls, bring 1 inch of water to a boil in a large skillet. Trim asparagus spears to no longer than 6 inches. Add asparagus to the boiling water. Partially cover and cook the asparagus until tender-crisp, about 3 minutes. Drain and refresh under cold water. Cut each spear in half lengthwise. Cut salmon slices into 12 strips no longer than 6 inches each. Soak one rice-paper wrapper at a time in a shallow dish of very hot water until softened, about 30 seconds. Lift out, let excess water drip off and lay on a clean, dry cutting board.

Center a strip of smoked salmon in the bottom third of the wrapper, leaving a 1-inch border on either side. Arrange 4 asparagus spear halves over the salmon. Top the asparagus with 2 avocado slices, 1 tablespoon shredded carrot and about 2 teaspoons each of basil and mint. Fold the wrapper over the filling and roll into a tight cylinder, folding in the ends as you go. Repeat with the remaining wrappers and filling. Cut each finished roll in half.

To prepare dipping sauce, whisk soy sauce, orange juice, lemon juice, mirin, and crushed red pepper in a small serving bowl. Serve the rolls with the sauce.

To make ahead: Individually wrap in parchment or wax paper and refrigerate for up to 4 hours.

BEEF BROCCOLI SALAD

Makes 4 servings

4 ounces uncooked wheat pasta linguine

Cooking spray

½ pound sirloin beef cut into chunks*

1½ cups broccoli florets

2 tablespoons cold water

5 green onions, sliced or chopped

1 cup chopped red bell pepper

¼ cup reduced-fat creamy peanut butter

2 tablespoons hot water

2 tablespoons low-sodium soy sauce

Dash of red pepper

Dash of garlic powder

1½ tablespoons extra-virgin olive or canola oil

½ cup unsalted peanuts, chopped

Cook pasta according to package directions. Drain and set aside. Spray a large nonstick skillet with cooking spray, add beef, and cook until no longer pink. Remove meat from skillet. Add broccoli and cold water to skillet. Cover and cook until broccoli is crisp-tender, approximately 3 to 5 minutes. Remove from skillet and combine pasta, meat, broccoli, onions, and pepper in a large bowl. In a small bowl, combine peanut butter, hot water, soy sauce, red pepper, and garlic powder, and use whisk to blend well. Add the oil gradually until combined to be smooth. Drizzle mixture over pasta and top with peanuts before serving.

*You can substitute chicken if you don't like beef.

BLACK BEAN PITA BURGERS

Makes 2 servings

2 cans black beans, rinsed
4 tablespoons fat-free mayo
¾ cup chopped cilantro
3 tablespoons dried bread crumbs
1½ teaspoons ground cumin
¾ teaspoon hot pepper sauce
Flour
2 small pita pockets or 1 large pita cut in half
Salsa
Lettuce
Tomato

Using potato masher, mash beans with mayo until smooth with some clumps. Mix cilantro, bread crumbs, cumin, and hot pepper sauce with the bean mixture. Flour hands and shape two cakes. Grill or pan fry patties for about 5 minutes on each side. Serve in pitas with salsa, lettuce, and tomato.

BUFFALO CHICKEN SALAD

Makes 4 servings

4 chicken breasts
½ cup buffalo sauce
¼ cup low-fat ranch dressing
1 large container salad lettuce
1 small cucumber, peeled, seeded, and chopped
½ cup sliced radishes
1 large green or colored bell pepper
1 cup sliced carrots
1 cup snap peas
One 8-ounce container cherry tomatoes
2 hard-boiled eggs, peeled and chopped
½ cup low-fat cheddar cheese

Grill or bake chicken breasts. After allowing them to cool, cut chickn into strips. Mix buffalo sauce and ranch dressing together in a small bowl. Add chicken and toss to coat. Combine lettuce with the other vegetables and the eggs. Top with chicken and cheddar cheese.

CALIFORNIA CHICKEN DINNER SALAD

Serves 6

3 bags of prewashed fresh mixed baby greens
2 cups shredded rotisserie chicken
1 bundle of 8–10 green onions, chopped
½ cup chopped fresh cilantro
½ cup chopped Italian parsley
3 tablespoons of fresh rosemary, chopped
One 15-ounce can garbanzo beans, drained and washed
1 bell pepper, any color, chopped
6 Medjool dates, pitted and diced
6 celery sticks, chopped
1 box/package of mushrooms, any kind, chopped
½ cup chopped raw nuts, any kind
⅓ cup raw sunflower seeds
⅓ cup low-fat cheese of your choice, crumbled or shredded
1 avocado, diced
½ teaspoon salt
½ teaspoon pepper
1 lemon
1 small orange

Combine ingredients in large salad bowl, starting with the greens and working your way through the pepper. Squeeze the juice of the lemon and orange onto the salad and mix thoroughly. Top with low-fat or nonfat salad dressing of choice.

CHICKEN BERRY SALAD

Makes 4 servings

- ¼ cup cider vinegar
- ½ cup vegetable oil
- 1 ounce honey mustard
- 2 tablespoons orange juice
- 1 pound skinless, boneless chicken breast halves
- 8 cups mixed salad greens
- 1 cup sliced fresh strawberries
- ½ cup fresh blueberries
- ½ cup fresh raspberries
- 8 ounces sugar snap peas
- ½ cup toasted pecans

In a medium bowl, whisk together vinegar, oil, honey mustard, and orange juice to create dressing. Set aside. Preheat the grill and lightly oil the grill grate. Grill chicken 6 to 8 minutes on each side, or until juices run clear.* Remove from heat, let cool, and slice into strips. In a large bowl, toss together the chicken, salad greens, strawberries, blueberries, raspberries, peas, and pecans. Pour in the prepared dressing, and toss to coat.

*If you don't have a grill, you can cook the chicken by broiling it on high heat until juices run clear.

CHICKEN PARMESAN

Makes 4 servings

3 tablespoon extra-virgin olive oil

2 cups cherry tomatoes, halved

½ cup basil, chopped

½ cup sliced shallots

Pepper to taste

½ cup dried whole-wheat bread crumbs

¼ cup grated Parmesan cheese

4 boneless, skinless chicken breasts

Heat 1 tablespoon oil in a skillet over medium-high heat. Add tomatoes, basil, shallots, and pepper, and cook for 10 minutes, stirring often. Remove from heat but cover to keep vegetable mixture warm. On a plate, mix bread crumbs with 2 tablespoons of Parmesan cheese and coat each chicken breast with bread-crumb mixture. Transfer coated chicken to a larger plate. In another skillet heat the other 2 tablespoons oil and add chicken, cook until golden brown and cooked through, approximately 5 to 6 minutes on each side. Spoon the vegetable mixture onto the chicken, and sprinkle with remaining Parmesan cheese, letting the cheese melt before serving.

CHICKEN TORTILLA SOUP

Makes 4 servings

4 boneless, skinless chicken breasts, chopped

4 ounces chopped green chilies, canned

2 tablespoons minced garlic

1 yellow onion, chopped

One 8-ounce can of black beans

One 8-ounce can of diced tomatoes

1 tablespoon ground cumin

2 tablespoons cilantro, chopped

2 cups water

1 fajita seasoning packet

4 corn tortillas sliced into ¼-inch strips for garnish

4 tablespoons fat-free sour cream or low-fat cheese (optional)

Combine first ten ingredients in a slow cooker and cook for 6 to 8 hours on medium heat. Separate into four bowls, and garnish with tortilla strips and sour cream or cheese, if desired.

CHICKEN WITH CARIBBEAN SALSA

Makes 4 servings

2 kiwifruits, peeled and chopped

1 cup chopped mango

½ cup chopped avocado

1 tablespoon lime juice

4 skinless, boneless chicken breast halves

1 teaspoon salt

½ teaspoon black pepper

1 tablespoon olive oil

½ teaspoon cumin seeds

1 onion, any color, chopped

2 bell peppers (red/yellow), diced

1 fresh jalapeño, stemmed, seeded, and cut into thin strips

2 cloves garlic, minced

¼ cup snipped fresh cilantro

In a medium bowl, combine kiwifruits, mango, avocado, and lime juice. Cover and set aside. Place one chicken breast half between two sheets of plastic wrap. Using the flat side of a meat mallet, pound chicken to ½-inch thickness. Repeat with remaining chicken breast halves. Remove chicken from plastic wrap and sprinkle each piece with ¼ teaspoon salt and ⅛ teaspoon black pepper.

In a large nonstick skillet, heat oil over a medium heat. Add chicken and cook until it is no longer pink, approximately 4 to 5 minutes on each side. Remove chicken from skillet, cut into slices, and keep warm. Add cumin seeds to the hot skillet, and cook until fragrant, about 30 seconds. Add onion, peppers, jalapeño, and garlic. Cook and stir until heated through, about 3 minutes. Stir in cilantro.

Divide pepper mixture among four plates. Top each with one sliced chicken breast half. Spoon mango mixture over chicken.

CRAB CAKE BURGERS

Makes 4 servings

1 pound crabmeat*
½ cup Egg Beaters or other egg substitute
½ cup panko bread crumbs
¼ cup fat-free mayo
2 tablespoons minced chives
1 tablespoon Dijon mustard
1 tablespoon lemon juice
1 teaspoon celery seed
1 teaspoon onion powder
¼ teaspoon ground pepper
4 dashes Tabasco
2 teaspoons unsalted butter, room temperature
1 tablespoon extra-virgin olive oil
4 large lettuce leaves

Pulse crabmeat in the food processor a couple times, or manually shred using a fork and spoon. Combine crabmeat, Egg Beaters, bread crumbs, mayo, chives, mustard, lemon juice, celery seed, onion powder, pepper, and Tabasco in large bowl. Add butter and mix all ingredients thoroughly. Heat olive oil in skillet. Brown crab cakes. Serve on lettuce leaves.

*You can substitute rotisserie chicken if you don't like crabmeat.

CURRIED CHICKEN

Makes 4 servings

4 cups cooked brown rice
1 rotisserie chicken, shredded or torn into small pieces
One 12-ounce can garbanzo beans
1 can hot Rotel
1 can mild Rotel
1 cup fat-free sour cream
¼ teaspoon each of salt, pepper, curry powder, and cumin

Prepare rice following directions on package. Meanwhile, in large pot, combine chicken, beans, Rotel, and sour cream. Add spices. Heat on medium-high, until bubbling, then reduce heat to low and simmer for 20 minutes. Serve over brown rice.

FISH TACOS

Makes 4 servings

Topping:
¼ cup thinly sliced green onions
¼ cup chopped fresh cilantro
3 tablespoons fat-free mayo
3 tablespoons reduced-fat sour cream
1 teaspoon grated lime rind
1½ teaspoons fresh lime juice
¼ teaspoon salt
1 garlic clove, minced

Tacos:
1 teaspoon ground cumin
1 teaspoon ground coriander
½ teaspoon smoked paprika
¼ teaspoon ground red pepper
⅛ teaspoon garlic powder
1½ pounds red snapper fillets
Cooking spray
8 (6-inch) corn tortillas
2 cups shredded cabbage

Preheat oven to 425 degrees. To prepare topping, combine topping ingredients in small bowl; set aside. To prepare tacos, combine spices in a small bowl, then sprinkle spice mixture evenly over both sides of fish. Place fish on a baking sheet coated with cooking spray. Bake for 10 minutes or until fish flakes easily when tested with a fork. Place fish in a bowl and break into pieces using a fork. Heat tortillas according to package directions. Divide fish evenly among tortillas and top each with ¼ cup cabbage and 1 tablespoon topping.

GREEK STUFFED PEPPERS

Makes 4 servings

4 yellow, orange, and/or red bell peppers
½ cup whole-wheat orzo
One 15-ounce can chickpeas, rinsed
1 tablespoon extra-virgin olive oil
1 medium onion, any color, chopped
6 ounces baby spinach, coarsely chopped
1 tablespoon chopped fresh oregano or 1 teaspoon dried
¾ cup crumbled fat-free feta cheese, divided
¼ cup sun-dried tomatoes (not oil-packed), chopped
1 tablespoon red-wine vinegar
¼ teaspoon salt

Halve peppers lengthwise through stems leaving stem on. Remove seeds and membranes. Place peppers, cut side down, in a microwave-safe dish with ½ inch water. Cover and heat in microwave on high for 7 to 9 minutes. Let cool, drain, and set aside. Cook orzo according to package directions, then drain and rinse with cold water. Mash chickpeas into a chunky paste, leaving some whole. Heat oil in skillet over medium heat. Add onion and cook until soft, about 4 minutes. Add spinach and oregano and cook until spinach is wilted, about 1 minute. Stir in orzo, chickpeas, ½ cup of feta, tomatoes, vinegar, and salt. Cook until heated through, about 1 minute. Divide filling between the pepper halves and sprinkle each with the remaining feta.

KABOBS

Makes 4 servings

- 2 tricolored bell peppers, cubed
- 1 onion, sliced
- 1 pineapple, cubed
- 2 chicken breasts, cubed
- 2 chicken apple sausages, cubed

Marinate the peppers, onion, and pineapple in low-sodium teriyaki sauce for 1 hour. Skewer chicken, sausages, peppers, onion, and pineapple. Preheat the grill* for high heat. Lightly oil the grill grate. Grill the chicken 6 to 8 minutes on each side, or until juices run clear.

*If you don't have a grill, you can cook skewers in a skillet.

LETTUCE WRAPS

Makes 6 servings

Sauce:
½ cup hoisin sauce
½ cup pomegranate juice
1 teaspoon sugar
1 teaspoon grated orange rind

Filling:
4 cups coleslaw mix or broccoli slaw mix
1 medium jalapeño pepper, seeded and sliced thinly
¼ cup chopped cilantro
1½ cups frozen edamame, thawed
1 cup matchstick carrots
3 boneless chicken breasts, cooked and diced

12 Bibb lettuce leaves or romaine leaves
2 ounces toasted peanuts

Combine sauce ingredients in small bowl and set aside. Combine filling ingredients. Arrange lettuce leaves on large serving platter. Spoon about ⅓ cup mixture on top of each leaf, drizzle sauce on top, and sprinkle with peanuts.

MEATBALL MARINARA

Makes 4 servings

Meatballs:
1½ pounds ground turkey
1 tablespoon Italian seasoning
1 egg
¼ cup grated Parmesan cheese
½ cup whole-wheat bread crumbs
1 tablespoon chopped parsley

Sauce:
1 tablespoon extra-virgin olive oil
4 cloves garlic, chopped
Two 14-ounce cans crushed tomatoes
½ teaspoon red pepper flakes
1 cup low-sodium chicken stock
½ teaspoon salt
½ teaspoon pepper

4 whole-grain sandwich rolls
1 cup shredded part-skim mozzarella

To make the meatballs, preheat oven to 425 degrees. Place turkey in a large bowl and add Italian seasoning, egg, Parmesan, bread crumbs, and parsley. Mix to combine, then form 20 one-inch meatballs. Bake for 15 minutes until golden brown.

To make sauce, heat large pot over medium heat. Add oil, garlic, tomatoes, red pepper, and chicken stock. Season with salt and pepper.

Add cooked meatballs to sauce. Place 5 meatballs on toasted sub roll. Sprinkle each sandwich with ¼ cup cheese.

MEDITERRANEAN BAKED FISH

Makes 4 servings

2 teaspoons extra-virgin olive oil

1 large onion, any color, sliced

One 16-ounce can whole tomatoes, drained (reserve juice) and coarsely chopped

1 bay leaf

1 clove garlic, minced

¾ cup apple juice

½ cup reserved tomato juice, from canned tomatoes

¼ cup lemon juice

¼ cup orange juice

1 tablespoon fresh grated orange peel

1 teaspoon fennel seeds, crushed

½ teaspoon dried oregano, crushed

½ teaspoon dried thyme, crushed

½ teaspoon dried basil, crushed

½ teaspoon black pepper

1 pound fish fillets (sole, flounder, or sea perch)

Preheat oven to 375 degrees. Heat oil in large nonstick skillet. Add onion, and sauté over moderate heat 5 minutes or until soft. Add all remaining ingredients except fish. Stir well and simmer 30 minutes, uncovered. Arrange fish in 10" x 6" baking dish; cover with sauce. Bake, uncovered, for about 15 minutes or until fish flakes easily.

MINI PIZZA

Makes 1 serving

½ 100% whole-wheat thin buns
1 tablespoon pizza sauce
½ cup thinly sliced veggies
¼ cup shredded part-skim mozzarella cheese

Preheat oven to 350 degrees. Toast bun in oven until slightly brown. Top with pizza sauce, veggies, and cheese. Bake in oven until cheese is melted.

OPEN-FACE BAGEL MELT

Makes 1 serving

½ 100% whole-wheat bagel thin
2-3 slices low-sodium deli turkey
½ tablespoon Dijon mustard
½ cup thinly sliced veggies
1 slice reduced-fat Swiss cheese

Preheat oven to 350 degrees. Toast bagel thin in oven until slightly brown. Add turkey breast, mustard, then veggies, and cheese. Bake in oven until cheese is melted.

PULLED PORK WITH CARAMELIZED ONIONS

Makes 10 servings

1 tablespoon extra-virgin olive oil

3 large onions, thinly sliced

⅓ cup raw cane sugar, such as demerara or turbinado

4 cloves garlic, minced

1 teaspoon dried oregano

1 teaspoon freshly ground pepper

½ teaspoon salt

⅓ cup cider vinegar

1 cup chili sauce

1½ –3 teaspoons minced chipotle chile in adobo sauce

3 pounds boneless pork shoulder or blade roast, trimmed

Heat oil in a large skillet over medium-high heat. Add onions and cook, stirring occasionally, until they begin to soften, approximately 3 to 6 minutes. Add sugar and continue to cook, stirring constantly, until the onions are golden brown, about 6 to 8 minutes more. Stir in garlic, oregano, pepper, and salt, and cook, stirring, for 1 minute. Add vinegar and bring to a boil, cooking until mostly evaporated, approximately 30 seconds to 1 minute. Remove from heat and stir in chili sauce and chipotle to taste. Place pork in a 4-quart slow cooker and cover with the sauce. Cover and cook until the pork is almost falling apart, about 4 hours on high or 8 hours on low. Transfer the pork to a cutting board and shred using two forks. Stir back into the sauce.

SAUTÉED PORK CHOPS WITH APPLES

Makes 4 servings

Four 8-ounce bone-in center-cut pork chops, cut ¾-inch thick

1 tablespoon plus 2 teaspoons canola oil

1 tablespoon Sugar and Spice Rub*

¼ cup dry white wine

2 cups thinly sliced Granny Smith apples

½ cup reduced-sodium chicken broth

1 sprig fresh thyme

Trim fat from chops. Brush 2 teaspoons oil over all sides of chops. Sprinkle chops evenly with Sugar and Spice Rub, and rub in with your fingers. Cover chops with plastic wrap and chill in refrigerator 1 hour. Preheat a large skillet over medium-high heat for 2 minutes. Add 1 tablespoon oil, swirling to lightly coat skillet. Add chops and cook until golden brown and juices run clear, approximately 5 to 6 minutes on each side. Transfer chops to a warm platter and cover to keep warm. Remove skillet from heat. Slowly add wine to hot skillet, stirring to scrape up browned bits from bottom of skillet. Return skillet to heat. Add apples, broth, and thyme. Bring to boiling; then reduce heat. Simmer, covered, about 3 minutes or until apples are tender. Using a slotted spoon, transfer apples to a small bowl; cover to keep warm. Bring broth mixture in skillet to boiling. Boil until liquid is reduced by half, about 5 minutes. Return chops and apples to skillet and heat through. Serve immediately.

Sugar and Spice Rub: In a small bowl, stir together 2 tablespoons brown sugar; 2 teaspoons chili powder; 1½ teaspoons each kosher salt, garlic powder, onion powder, and ground cumin; and ¾ teaspoon each cayenne pepper and black pepper. Store in an airtight container up to 3 months. Makes about ½ cup rub.

SLOW-COOKER POT ROAST

Makes 4 servings

1 pound of rump roast
2 cloves garlic, chopped
2 teaspoons ground pepper
4 large carrots, chopped
1 large onion, any color, coarsely chopped
1 tablespoon rosemary
1 tablespoon thyme
1 tablespoon black pepper
½ cup low-sodium soy sauce

In a slow cooker, cover meat with the rest of the ingredients, then add enough water to cover the roast. Cook on low heat for 6 to 8 hours.

SOUTHWEST TURKEY BAKE

Makes 4 servings

1 pound extra-lean ground turkey
1 can black beans, rinsed
1 cup salsa
½ teaspoon cumin
⅛ teaspoon ground red pepper
One 8–12-ounce package corn muffin mix
¾ cup reduced-sodium chicken broth
⅓ cup Egg Beaters or other egg substitute
¾ cup reduced-fat shredded Mexican cheese

Preheat oven to 400 degrees. Brown turkey in a skillet, then add black beans, salsa, cumin, and red pepper and simmer for 2 minutes. Layer turkey mixture on bottom of 13" x 9"-inch baking dish. In a medium bowl, combine corn muffin mix, broth, and Egg Beaters and stir well. Spread corn-muffin mixture over turkey to cover and sprinkle with cheese. Bake 15 minutes or until edges are lightly browned.

SPICY TUNA WRAP

Makes 4 servings

Two 6-ounce cans chunk light tuna in water, drained
⅓ cup fat-free mayo
1 tablespoon hot sauce, such as Sriracha
1 scallion, chopped
1 cup cooked brown rice, cooled
2 tablespoons rice vinegar
Four 10-inch whole-grain or whole-wheat wraps
3 cups watercress leaves
1 ripe avocado, cut into 16 slices
1 small carrot, cut into matchsticks
Soy sauce (optional)

Combine tuna, mayo, hot sauce, and scallion in a medium bowl. Combine rice and vinegar in a small bowl. Spread one-fourth of the tuna mixture over a wrap. Top with one quarter of the rice, watercress, avocado, and carrot matchsticks. Roll up and cut the wrap in quarters or in half. Repeat with the remaining filling and wraps. Serve with soy sauce for dipping, if desired.

SUMMER JAMBALAYA

Makes 6 servings

1 package spicy jalapeño chicken sausage
1 tablespoon olive oil
2 tablespoons sherry dry
1 cup fresh salsa
2 cups mango chunks
1 cup pineapple chunks in own juice
1 cup prepared fresh/frozen edamame
1 cup black beans
2 tablespoons cilantro
3 cups cooked brown rice

Cut sausages into bite-size pieces and sauté for approximately 15 minutes in olive oil over high heat. Add sherry and cook 2 minutes. In small bowl, mix fresh salsa with the mango and pineapple. Add the salsa mix, edamame, and black beans to sausage pan. Continue to cook until bubbling. Remove from heat. Chop cilantro and mix it with the rice. Spoon the sausage mix over the rice, then serve.

TACOS

Makes 4 servings

8 tostadas (whole corn)
1 cup low-fat refried black beans
12 ounces rotisserie chicken, shredded white meat
1 ripe avocado, peeled, pitted, and diced
4 tablespoons fat-free sour cream
1 cup romaine lettuce, chopped
1 cup chunky salsa

Preheat oven to 350 degrees. Arrange tostadas on baking sheet in a single layer and bake for 3 to 5 minutes. Meanwhile mix beans and chicken and heat on stove over medium-high until warmed through. Spread tostadas with bean-and-chicken mixture, then top with avocado, sour cream, lettuce, and salsa.

WHITE BEAN CHICKEN CHILI

Makes 2 servings

1 tablespoon vegetable oil
½ onion, any color, chopped
1 clove garlic, minced
8 ounces chicken broth
One 8-ounce can tomatillos, chopped
One 8-ounce can diced tomatoes
4 ounces diced green chiles
¼ teaspoon oregano
¼ teaspoon coriander seed
⅛ teaspoon ground cumin
1 ear fresh corn or ½ cup canned corn
1½ cups cooked chicken, diced
One 8-ounce can white beans, rinsed

In large pan, heat oil and cook onion and garlic until soft. Stir in broth, tomatillos, tomatoes, chiles, and spices. Bring to a boil over high heat, and simmer 10 minutes. Add corn, chicken, and beans. Simmer 5 minutes.

Appendix D

THE FULL DIET
SNACK IDEAS

Snack Guidelines:

- All snacks should contain 5–14 gm protein per serving.

- Do not exceed 200 calories per serving.

Single Item Snacks:

Choose one item; add vegetable serving if desired.

- Any Fullbar product (100–200 calories/5–10 gm protein)

- 1 ounce nuts (167 calories/6 gm protein)

- 4 ounces low-fat Greek yogurt (130 calories/11 gm protein)

- ¼ cup hummus (102 calories/5 gm protein)

- 2 tablespoons low-fat peanut butter (146 calories/7 gm protein)

- 1 ounce beef jerky (115 calories/9 gm protein)

- ½ cup edamame, shelled (100 calories/8 gm protein)

Double Item Snacks:

Protein Choices:

Combine 1 Protein Choice + 1 Carbohydrate Choice = 1 Snack Serving

- 1 ounce low-fat cheese (48 calories/7 gm protein)
- 2 ounces fat-free cream cheese (58 calories/8 gm protein)
- ¼ cup low-fat cottage cheese (81 calories/14 gm protein)
- ½ cup fat-free refried beans (90 calories/6 gm protein)
- 2 ounces reduced-sodium lean deli meat (60 calories/12 gm protein)
- 6 ounces Dannon Light & Fit Yogurt (80 calories/5 gm protein)
- 1 hard-boiled egg (77 calories/7 gm protein)
- 1 ounce tuna (32 calories/7 gm protein)

Carbohydrate Choices:

- 1 cup celery sticks (16 calories)
- ½ cup carrots (52 calories)
- 1 cup green peppers (30 calories)
- 1 cup cucumbers (16 calories)
- 1 cup cherry tomatoes (27 calories)
- 10 Wheat Thin Fiber Selects (120 calories)
- ½ 100% whole-wheat English muffin (50 calories)
- ½ whole-wheat pita (85 calories)
- 1 cup berries: strawberries, blueberries, etc. (49 calories)

- 1 cup cantaloupe, honeydew, or watermelon (64 calories)

- ½ cup pineapple (41 calories)

- 1 cup grapes (62 calories)

- 1 small apple (53 calories)

Note: Nutritional values are approximate and dependent on brand and ripeness of produce.

Acknowledgments

It's true what they say: it takes a virtual army of bright, passionate people to put a book together. This one is no different. I owe everyone I've ever worked with and treated through the years a heartfelt thank-you. The unwavering support of my family, friends, and colleagues has paved the path to this book. Your guidance, insights, and feedback were indispensable; *Full* is as much yours as it is mine.

I owe my wife, Robin, more gratitude and appreciation than words can express—especially for enduring the moments I took away from her life and our family when I dashed out to treat a patient at dinnertime or answered a call in the middle of the night. Her relentless encouragement, faith in me, love, and wisdom always keep me inspired and focused. When she says things like, "You should go see that patient. You seem really worried," it is the reality check I need and treasure. And to our children, Eli and Sage, who have been gracious champions of my career and crazy life. They have not only tolerated having a multitasking dad, but gone beyond the call of duty—being constant sources of unconditional love and guidance. Their integrity, bravery, and beyond-their-years perspective have taught me far more than 24 years of school and training. I believe that they have ultimately taught me *all* of the critical stuff I need to know.

I would like to extend my profound gratitude to my loving parents who never quite knew what to do with me and my ideas. Whenever I doubted myself, they always reassured me with "You'll be fine." Ultimately, with the life and education they gave me, they were right.

When I first spoke with Bonnie Solow about doing a book, I knew it was finally time to share the knowledge I had been collecting through the years of my practice, much of which could be used to enhance the health of millions. Bonnie quickly saw the passion in me and embraced my philosophy. Thank you, Bonnie, for lighting the way and enabling me to finally reach those people. Your leadership and steadfast commitment to this project from its early stages have been invaluable.

Thank you, Kristin Loberg, my writing partner, who helped me get what I needed to say down in writing. Keeping the layman's ear in mind, she helped me craft what I hope is a compelling and convincing message about how you can take charge of your weight in ways you never thought possible. I cannot say that I will miss our marathon, four-day weekend, sixteen-hour daily writing sessions (or my constant writing assignments)—but they were certainly memorable and important.

I will forever be indebted to the team at Fullbar, Inc., whose loyal support and creative marketing genius make my job easier and the delivery of my message to the world possible. You know who you are. Thanks for always keeping me on track and for helping me balance my roles as a physician, an entrepreneur, and a zealous defender of those trapped in the weight-control struggle. I owe a special thanks to my Fullbar business partner, Joel Appel. Without his trust in my vision, faith in my potential, and unbridled love of the process, the idea of this book would never have been entertained. Together, we have certainly tested the limits of what it means to be friends and in business together. And I am always amazed at how well things turn out with Joel at my side.

To my team at The Denver Center for Bariatric Surgery and Rose Medical Center. From my office staff, to the bariatric program specialists, to the 6th-floor nurses, to my OR Room #4 team—your tireless support of our patients and love of what you do make my day-to-day life so much more complete. Your commitment to our patients' safety and humanity on every level are what makes our program a worldwide leader in the field of bariatric surgery.

To my publishing stewards at Hay House, especially Louise Hay, Reid Tracy, Patty Gift, Laura Koch, Sally Mason, Margarete Nielsen, Jeannie Liberati, Lindsay McGinty, and Richelle Zizian. Your enthusiasm and leadership in the publishing process have made for a sharper piece of work that speaks to a wide audience.

And last, but certainly not least, I again wish to pay tribute to my patients. Honest, hardworking, and heroes of sheer dedication, they are the ones who keep me on my toes; who nurture me into a more thoughtful, better doctor; and who help me try to make the world a healthier place . . . one individual at a time.

About the Author

Michael A. Snyder, M.D., F.A.C.S., is a board-certified general surgeon and a highly respected leader and mentor in the field of bariatric surgery. He has performed more than 2,700 primary bariatric surgical procedures including postsurgical coaching and ongoing health care. Snyder is a Fellow of the American College of Surgeons and founder of The Denver Center for Bariatric Surgery, a comprehensive, state-of-the-art surgical practice specializing in weight loss. He also is the founder of Fullbar, LLC, a multimillion-dollar company dedicated to improving the quality of people's lives and helping them achieve their weight-loss goals through food products that assist them in feeling full so they eat less.

A tireless crusader for health and wellness, Dr. Snyder is deeply passionate about helping people lose weight and live healthier, happier, and *fuller* lives. His mission is straightforward: to simplify weight loss by helping people feel full so they eat less. He wants to add to people's lives—not take away from them.

Hay House Titles of Related Interest

YOU CAN HEAL YOUR LIFE, the movie,
starring Louise L. Hay & Friends
(available as a 1-DVD program and an expanded 2-DVD set)
Watch the trailer at: **www.LouiseHayMovie.com**

THE SHIFT, the movie,
starring Dr. Wayne W. Dyer
(available as a 1-DVD program and an expanded 2-DVD set)
Watch the trailer at: **www.DyerMovie.com**

∿

*THE BELLY FAT CURE™: Discover the New Carb Swap System
and Lose 4 to 9 lbs. Every Week,* by Jorge Cruise

*THE CORE BALANCE DIET: 4 Weeks to Boost Your Metabolism
and Lose Weight for Good,* by Marcelle Pick, MSN, OB/GYN NP

*A COURSE IN WEIGHT LOSS: 21 Spiritual Lessons for
Surrendering Your Weight Forever,* by Marianne Williamson

*LIGHTEN UP!: The Authentic and Fun Way to Lose Your
Weight and Your Worries,* by Loretta LaRoche

*THE RIGHT WEIGH: Six Steps to Permanent Weight Loss
Used by More Than 100,000 People,* by Rena Greenberg

*THE SPARK: The 28-Day Breakthrough Plan for Losing Weight,
Getting Fit, and Transforming Your Life,* by Chris Downie

All of the above are available at your local bookstore,
or may be ordered by contacting Hay House (see next page).

∿

We hope you enjoyed this Hay House book. If you'd like
to receive our online catalog featuring additional information
on Hay House books and products, or if you'd like to find
out more about the Hay Foundation, please contact:

Hay House, Inc., P.O. Box 5100, Carlsbad, CA 92018-5100
(760) 431-7695 or (800) 654-5126
(760) 431-6948 (fax) or (800) 650-5115 (fax)
www.hayhouse.com® • **www.hayfoundation.org**

Published and distributed in Australia by: Hay House Australia Pty.
Ltd., 18/36 Ralph St., Alexandria NSW 2015 • *Phone:* 612-9669-4299
Fax: 612-9669-4144 • www.hayhouse.com.au

Published and distributed in the United Kingdom by: Hay House UK,
Ltd., 292B Kensal Rd., London W10 5BE • *Phone:* 44-20-8962-1230
Fax: 44-20-8962-1239 • www.hayhouse.co.uk

Published and distributed in the Republic of South Africa by:
Hay House SA (Pty), Ltd., P.O. Box 990, Witkoppen 2068
Phone/Fax: 27-11-467-8904 • www.hayhouse.co.za

Published in India by: Hay House Publishers India,
Muskaan Complex, Plot No. 3, B-2, Vasant Kunj, New Delhi 110 070
Phone: 91-11-4176-1620 • *Fax:* 91-11-4176-1630 • www.hayhouse.co.in

Distributed in Canada by: Raincoast, 9050 Shaughnessy St.,
Vancouver, B.C. V6P 6E5 • *Phone:* (604) 323-7100
Fax: (604) 323-2600 • www.raincoast.com

Take Your Soul on a Vacation

Visit **www.HealYourLife.com®** to regroup, recharge, and reconnect
with your own magnificence. Featuring blogs, mind-body-spirit news,
and life-changing wisdom from Louise Hay and friends.

Visit **www.HealYourLife.com** today!

NOTES

NOTES